Hrayr P. Attarian • Nidhi S. Undevia

Atlas of Electroencephalography in Sleep Medicine

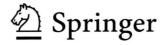 Springer

Hrayr P. Attarian
Division of Sleep Medicine
Department of Neurology
Northwestern University
Feinberg School of Medicine
Chicago, IL, USA
zeesmd@gmail.com

Nidhi S. Undevia
Division of Pulmonary & Critical Care Medicine
Department of Medicine
Loyola University Medical Center
Maywood, IL, USA
nundevia@lumc.edu

ISBN 978-1-4614-2292-1   e-ISBN 978-1-4614-2293-8
DOI 10.1007/978-1-4614-2293-8
Springer New York Dordrecht Heidelberg London

Library of Congress Control Number: 2011946069

To the memory of my father, Pierre Attarian. May it remain alive in the minds of the many people whose lives he touched.

Hrayr P. Attarian, M.D.

To my husband, Samir Undevia, and children, Akshay and Anisha, for their unwavering support.

Nidhi S. Undevia, M.D.

Preface

Sleep medicine is a diverse field that brings together the knowledge and expertise of a variety of medical specialties. This is easily demonstrated by the fact that the physicians who practice in this field come from a variety of backgrounds including internal medicine, otolaryngology, neurology, pediatrics, psychiatry, and pulmonary medicine. Despite our varied background, those of us practicing clinical sleep medicine find ourselves with very similar clinical practices regardless of our primary specialty. For those of us without neurology training, we have incorporated the review of sleep electroencephalograms (EEGs) into our daily lives, and those without pulmonary training have become more than familiar with oxygen desaturation, hypoventilation, and the use of supplemental oxygen.

There are, however, those instances in which gaps in knowledge can challenge the limits of our training. For those fortunate enough to work in multidisciplinary sleep programs with physicians with different primary specialties, I am sure that they have come to realize the benefits of collaboration and discussion in assisting both patient care and increasing the basic fund of knowledge.

It is out of the need to fill these gaps in knowledge where the idea for this book began. I am certain that many have had the experience when they are able to identify that something "is not right" or "looks different" about the EEG but are unable to identify the specific abnormality. As such, this book is intended for the sleep specialist without specific training in epileptology to assist with EEG interpretation during polysomnography review.

This book has been organized into five chapters. Chapters 1 and 2 focus on normal sleep, normal sleep stages and normal EEG variants in sleep, respectively. Chapter 3 focuses on non-epileptiform abnormalities, whereas Chap. 4 takes on epileptiform abnormalities. Chapter 5 reviews artifacts that may be seen on review of the EEG.

I would like to take a moment to comment on the layout of the figures in this book. All figures are real examples from patients studied in an epilepsy monitoring unit. Each example is shown as it would appear with channels recorded during routine polysomnography; however, the order of these channels has been changed to place the left-sided leads and right-sided leads together as is done in routine EEG monitoring. Current digital systems used for polysomnography allow the user to easily change the order of leads when indicated and can be helpful in the identification of EEG abnormalities. Subsequent figures show each topic with the full-EEG montage and then at the faster 30 mm/s paper speed used in EEG. Additional figures are shown, when appropriate, with reduced gains to demonstrate specific details about the topic in question.

It is our hope that readers will use this book to increase their knowledge regarding EEG findings in both normal and abnormal sleep and as an aid in polysomnography interpretation.

Chicago, IL, USA
Maywood, IL, USA

Hrayr P. Attarian, MD
Nidhi S. Undevia, MD

Acknowledgments

The authors would like to express their appreciation to Michael Macken, M.D., Rajinder Singh, D.O., and John Millichap, M.D., for their assistance in providing materials presented in this book, and to Ryan Hays, M.D., for critical review of some of the samples.

Our thanks are also extended to Lee Klein for his wonderful administrative assistance throughout the project.

Contents

Normal Sleep Stages

1

Keywords

Normal awake • Alpha activity • N1; poorly formed alpha activity • Vertex waves • Spindles • K complexes • Delta frequency slowing • Normal N3 • Normal R • Eye movement artifact • Sawtooth waves • Phasic R • Tonic R • Arousals

Wakefulness (Stage W): The "Alpha" Rhythm

Wakefulness (stage W) is characterized by the "alpha" rhythm, so named because it was the first electroencephalogram (EEG) rhythm discovered. Alpha frequency activity is 8–13 cycles/s and may be recorded anywhere in the brain. Alpha rhythm, however, has come to signify the sinusoidal resting rhythm of the occipital cortex. In addition to being in the above frequency range, it is usually of an amplitude around 30–50 mV and tends to occur in the posterior regions of the head, maximal over the occipital regions, and appears during relaxed wakefulness with eyes closed. In polysomnography interpretation, sleep onset is marked when the alpha rhythm attenuates and is absent from 50% of the epoch. The alpha rhythm, however, may attenuate and disappear when one is fully awake by just opening the eyes or thinking of a visual image. With sleep onset, the alpha frequency activity disappears not only from occipital channels but from all the electrodes (Figs. 1.1–1.6).

Stage N1 Sleep

The first stage of sleep for almost 90% of people who have well-formed alpha rhythms in relaxed wakefulness is characterized by the attenuation of posterior dominant activity together with overall slowing of the background for more than 50% of the epoch. For approximately 10% of people without the well-formed alpha rhythm, the overall slowing of background frequencies to theta (4–7 Hz) rhythm or a decrease by ≥1 Hz from stage W background activity with vertex waves and/or slow-rolling eye movements signifies the onset of N1 sleep [3] (Figs. 1.7–1.9).

N2 Sleep: Spindles and K Complexes

N2 sleep is characterized by low-amplitude, mixed-frequency background with two superimposed, morphologically distinct waveforms: sleep spindles and K complexes. The presence of either is necessary for scoring N2 [3].

A *sleep spindle* is defined as a series of distinct waves with frequency 11–16 Hz (commonly 12–14 Hz) with a duration ≥0.5 s, with the maximum amplitude usually over the central regions [3]. They often, but not always, are followed by a K complex. A K complex is a well-delineated negative sharp wave (upward deflection) immediately followed by a positive component (downward deflection), with total duration ≥0.5 s that stands out from the background EEG. It is usually maximal in amplitude over the frontal regions. K complexes can either be spontaneous or induced by a known sensory stimulus, although both look identical [3] (Figs. 1.10–1.15).

H.P. Attarian and N.S. Undevia, *Atlas of Electroencephalography in Sleep Medicine*, DOI 10.1007/978-1-4614-2293-8_1, © Springer Science+Business Media, LLC 2012

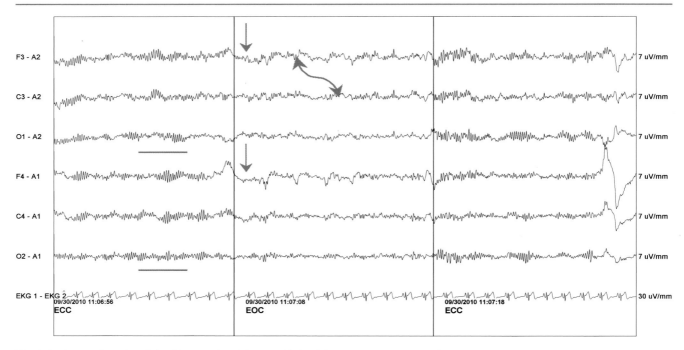

Fig. 1.1 A normal awake adult with eyes closed for two-thirds of the 30-s epoch. The high-frequency filter (HFF) is at 70 Hz and low-frequency filter (LFF) at 0.5 Hz. Notch filter is not on. *Blue lines* indicate where alpha activity is best seen. *Straight blue arrows* indicate the eye movement artifact as eyes open. *Curved arrows* show that, despite the disappearance of the alpha rhythm in the occipital channels, alpha frequency activity is present in other channels. ECC—eyes close command; EOC—eyes open command

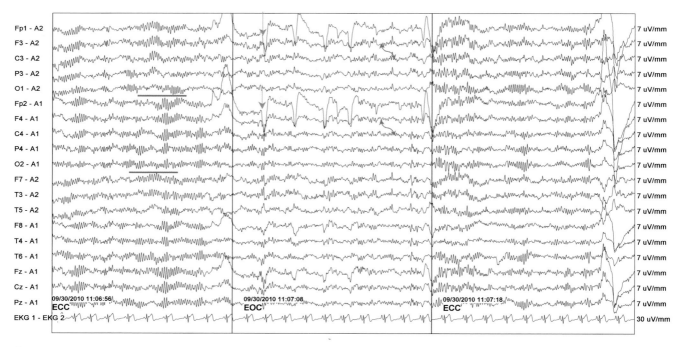

Fig. 1.2 The same epoch as in Fig. 1.1 but the alpha rhythm is now clearer on the 30-s epoch with extended EEG montage. *Blue lines* indicate where alpha activity is best seen. *Straight blue arrows* indicate the eye movement artifact as eyes open. *Curved arrows* show that, despite the disappearance of the alpha rhythm in the occipital channels, alpha frequency activity is present in other channels

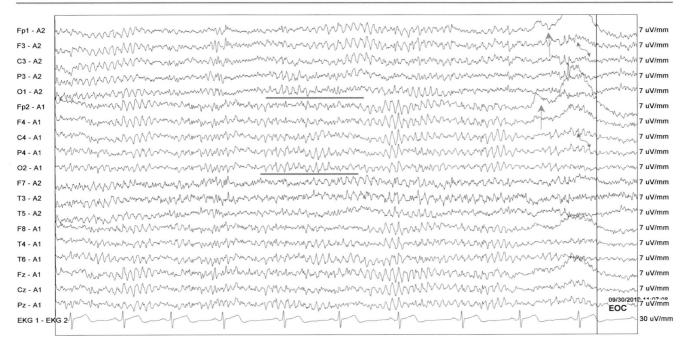

Fig. 1.3 A 10-s typical EEG epoch for the same patient as in Figs. 1.1 and 1.2

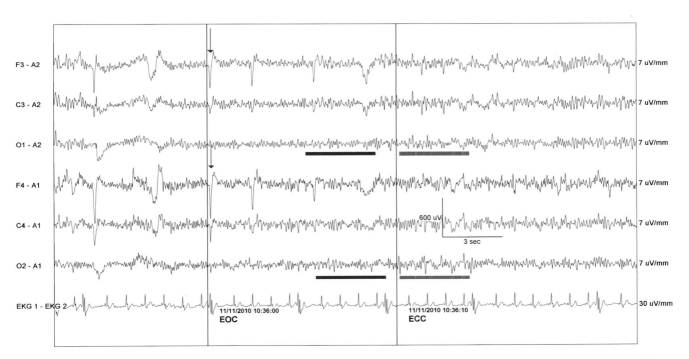

Fig. 1.4 A normal awake adult with eyes closed for two-thirds of the 30-s epoch. HFF is at 70 Hz and LFF at 0.5 Hz. Notch filter is not on. *Blue lines* indicate the absence of alpha activity because eyes are open. *Red lines* indicate points at which alpha rhythm reappears. *Straight blue arrows* indicate eye movement artifact as eyes open. The difference between eyes open and eyes closed is minimal on the occipital alpha rhythm, especially compared to Fig. 1.1. Sometimes alpha rhythm is poorly formed and less than clear. This occurs in approximately 10% of the population [1] and seems to be correlated with anxiety and emotional instability [2]

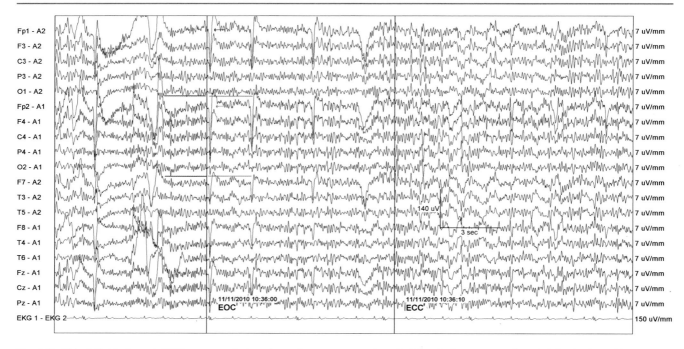

Fig. 1.5 This full 16-channel EEG montage derives from the same person as in Fig. 1.4. *Red arrows* indicate eye movement artifact when eyes open. *Blue lines* indicate poorly formed alpha rhythm before eye opening. *Red lines* indicate attenuation of alpha rhythm with eye opening. Although the difference is a bit clearer here, it is not as dramatic a difference as in Fig. 1.2

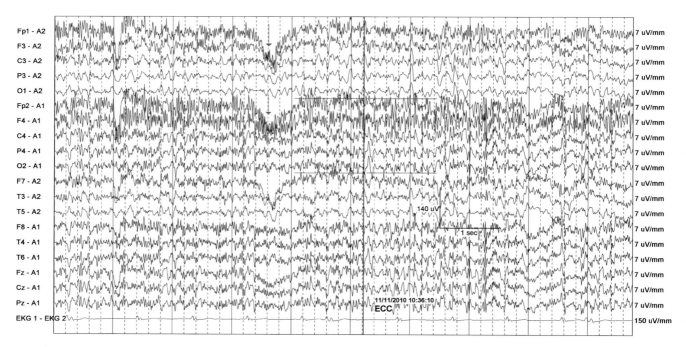

Fig. 1.6 A 10-s portion of the epoch in Fig. 1.5 demonstrates the same poorly formed occipital alpha activity. *Red arrows* indicate eye movement artifact when eyes close. *Red lines* indicate the absence of occipital rhythms when eyes open. *Green lines* indicate poorly formed alpha rhythm after eye closing

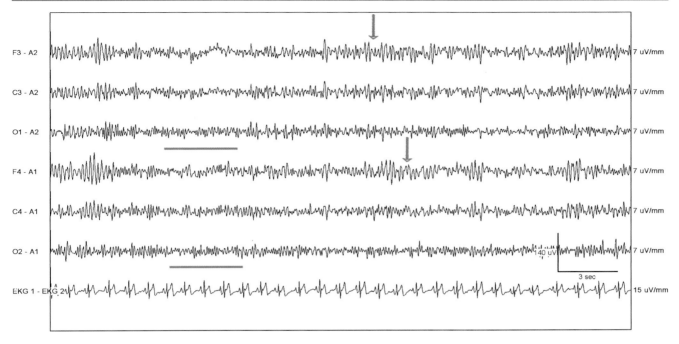

Fig. 1.7 Attenuation (*blue lines*) of the posterior dominant alpha rhythms, together with the prevalent theta slowing best seen in the frontal channels (*blue arrows*)

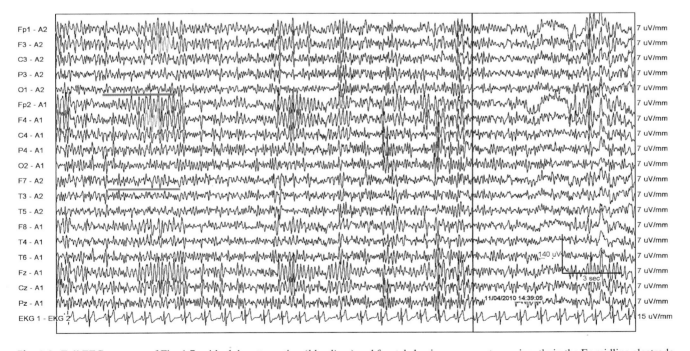

Fig. 1.8 Full EEG montage of Fig. 1.7, with alpha attenuation (*blue lines*) and frontal slowing seen most prominently in the Fz midline electrode (enhanced in *red*)

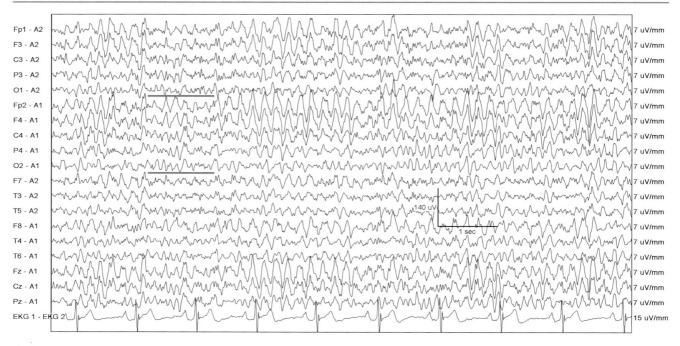

Fig. 1.9 A 10-s portion of the epoch as in Fig. 1.8

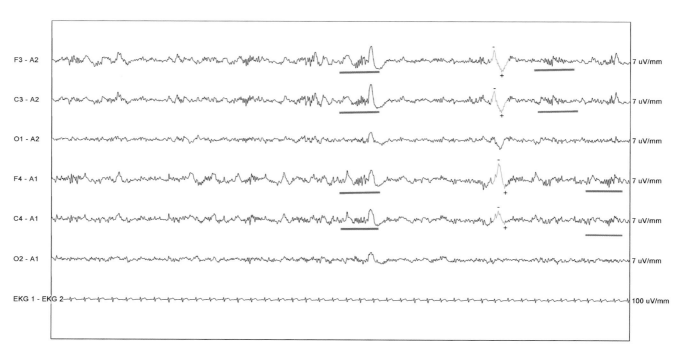

Fig. 1.10 Spindles (*blue lines*) and K complexes (enhanced in *red*), with negative and positive components marked

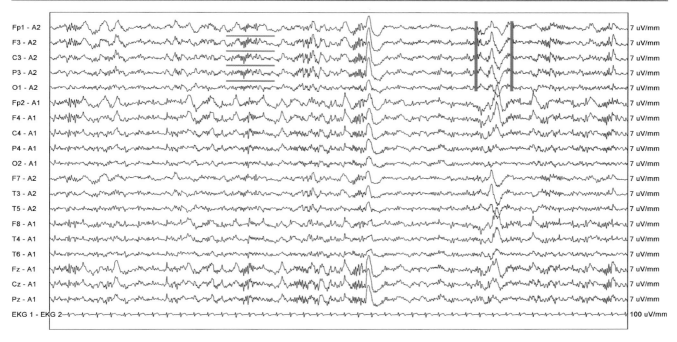

Fig. 1.11 Full EEG montage of Fig. 1.10 shows the K complex over the left parasagittal electrodes between the two *red bars*. It is obvious that the largest amplitude is at the F3 electrode, followed by C3. The spindles (*blue lines*), on the other hand, are equally well-defined in both F3 and C3

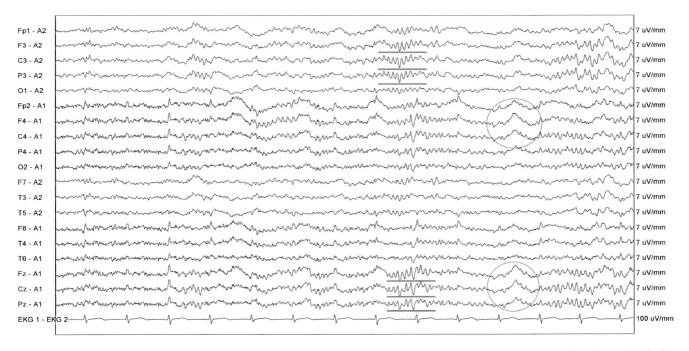

Fig. 1.12 This 10-s portion of the epoch as in Fig. 1.11 displaying the full EEG montage highlights K complexes (*red circles*) and spindles (*blue bars*)

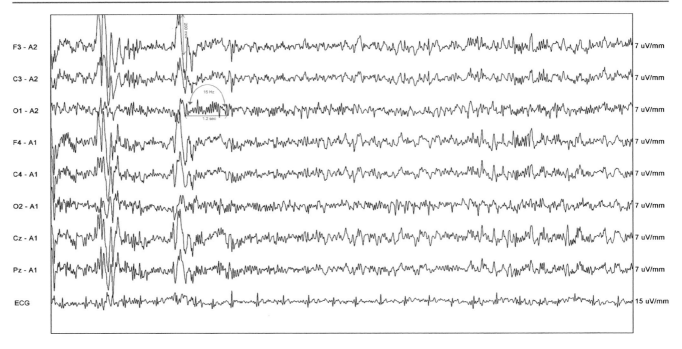

Fig. 1.13 In this 30-s epoch displaying a limited EEG, K complexes and spindles are clear and their duration (1.2 s), amplitude (200 mV), and frequency (15 Hz) are noted and highlighted

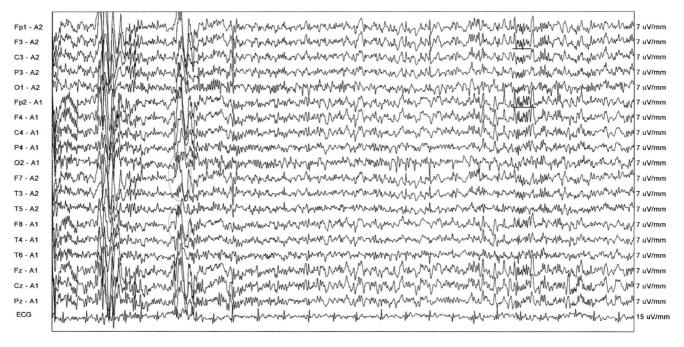

Fig. 1.14 The same epoch as in Fig. 1.13 but with an expanded EEG montage. *Red ovals* show K complexes and *blue lines* indicate spindles

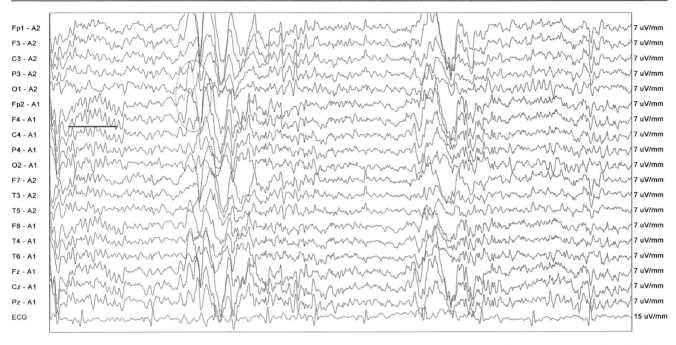

Fig. 1.15 The same patient as in Figs. 1.13 and 1.14 but this 10-s epoch displays a traditional EEG paper speed of 30 mm/s. The *red oval* indicates K complexes and the *blue line* indicates spindles

N3 Sleep: Frequency and Amplitude of Slow Waves

Formerly known as stage 3 and stage 4, or slow-wave sleep, N3 is a non-rapid eye movement (REM) sleep stage with the highest arousal threshold. It is characterized by high-amplitude (>75 mV) and slow-frequency (0.5–2 Hz) activity dominating ≥20% of the 30-s epoch. Of note, traditionally by EEG criteria, the slowest band is delta and the range is 0.5–4 Hz. Because N3 requires a frequency range of 0.5–2 Hz, to avoid confusion the term *delta sleep* should be discouraged [3] (Figs. 1.16–1.21).

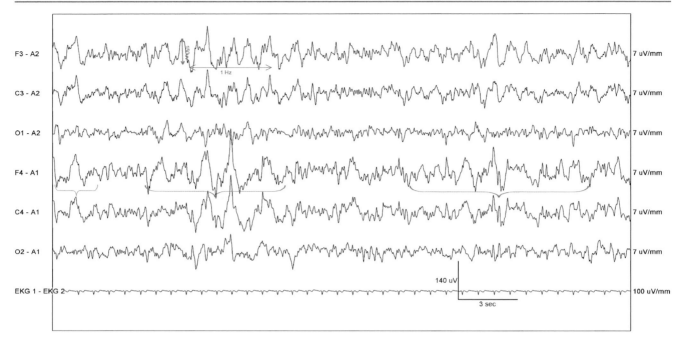

Fig. 1.16 The slow waves of 1 Hz and more than 75 mV in amplitude are bracketed in *red*. They are most prominent in the frontal channels, as expected

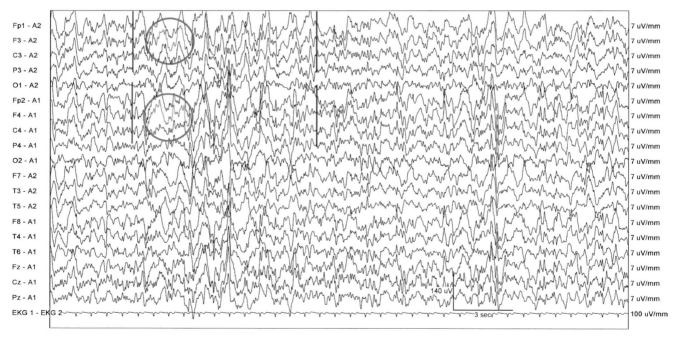

Fig. 1.17 The same epoch as in Fig. 1.16 but using a full EEG montage. *Red circles* highlight the individual waves and *blue lines* indicate the period of 10.5 s (35% of the epoch) dominated by these slow waves

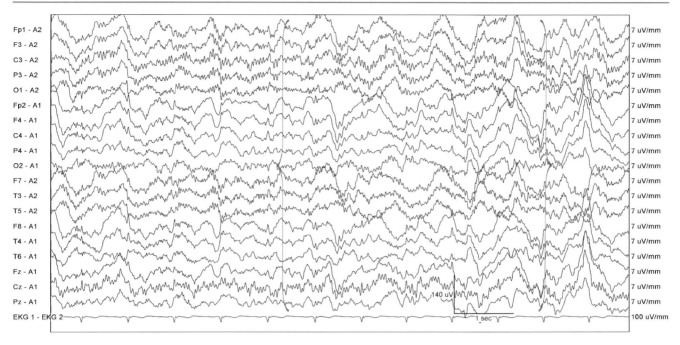

Fig. 1.18 The same epoch as in Fig. 1.17 but at the faster paper speed of traditional EEG. Each epoch is 10 s. *Red brackets* indicate slow waves

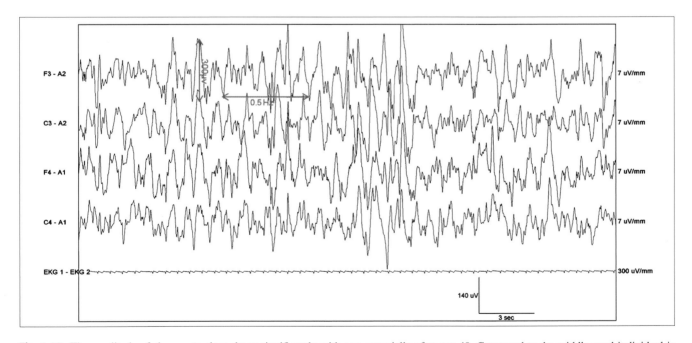

Fig. 1.19 The amplitude of slow-wave sleep drops significantly with age, especially after age 40. Compared to the middle-aged individual in Figs. 1.16 through 1.18, note how much higher the frequencies are in the N3 sleep of this teenager

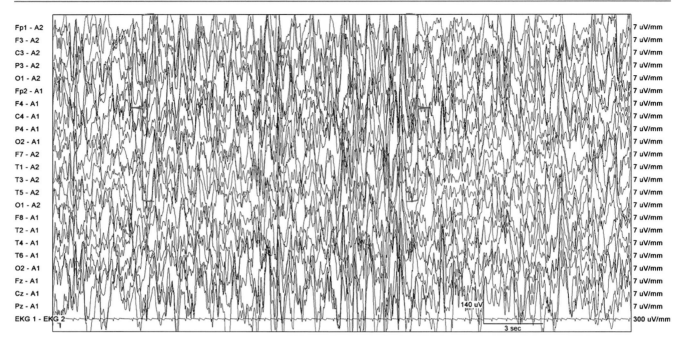

Fig. 1.20 The same epoch as in Fig. 1.19 but with a full EEG montage. *Red brackets* indicate the period with most slow-wave activity (about 50% of the epoch)

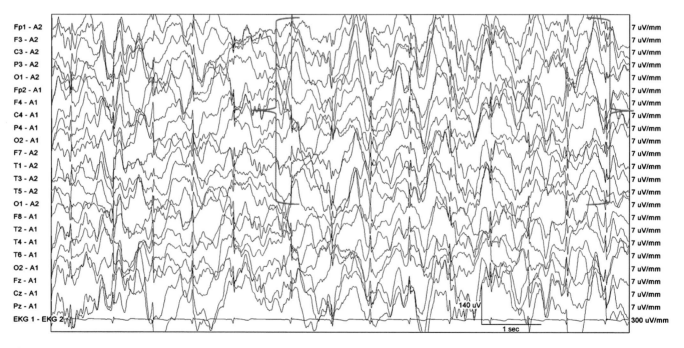

Fig. 1.21 Part of the same epoch as in Figs. 1.18 and 1.19 at the faster EEG speed of 30 mm/s is displayed, making the epoch length 10 s

Rapid Eye Movement Sleep (REM or Stage R)

According to the newer guidelines published in *The AASM Manual for the Scoring of Sleep and Associated Events* [4], the three essential electrographic phenomena required to score an epoch as stage R are (1) low amplitude and mixed frequency activity in the EEG channels, (2) presence of rapid eye movements, and (3) low muscle tone in the chin electromyogram (EMG) channel. Occasionally, an epoch can be scored as stage R without the presence of eye movements. Guidelines indicate that all epochs preceding and following a patient with clear eye movements can be scored as stage R if the chin tone remains low and there are no hallmarks of any other stage of sleep or wakefulness [3]. The epochs with the presence of eye movements occasionally accompanied by brief phasic twitching and sawtooth waves on EEG are known as *phasic REM* whereas intervening epochs without eye movements are known as *tonic REM* (Figs. 1.22–1.27).

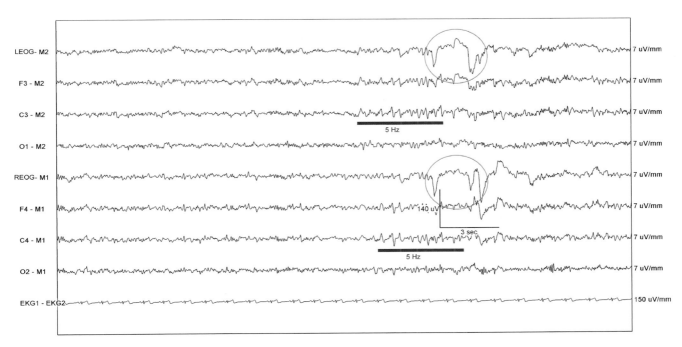

Fig. 1.22 A typical phasic REM period with eye movement (*circled in red*) fitting the determined criteria of irregular, sharply peaked eye movement with an initial deflection lasting less than 500 ms. Note also sawtooth waves (*underlined by blue bars*) on the EEG again fitting the criteria of sharply contoured, triangular, and serrated 2–6 Hz waves maximal over the central head regions and often preceding a burst of rapid eye movement

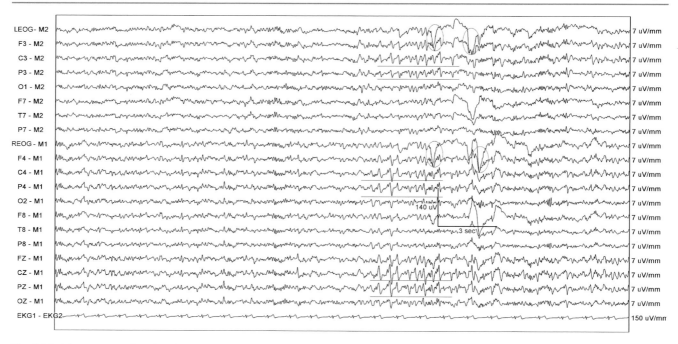

Fig. 1.23 The same epoch as in Fig. 1.22 but displaying a full EEG montage. Eye movements are *circled in red* and the sawtooth waves are *underlined in red*

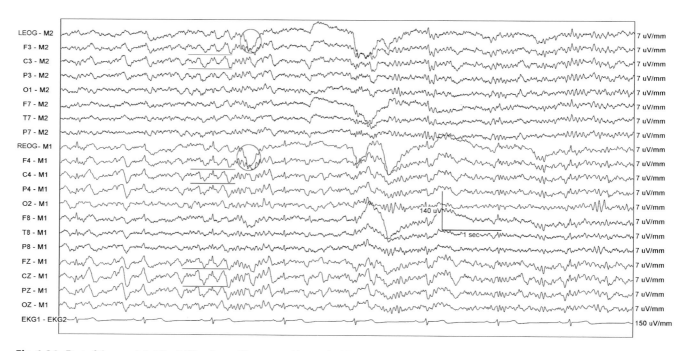

Fig. 1.24 Part of the epoch in Fig. 1.23 as it would appear with a typical EEG paper speed of 30 m/s resulting in 10-s epochs. Eye movements are *circled in red* and the sawtooth waves are *underlined in red*

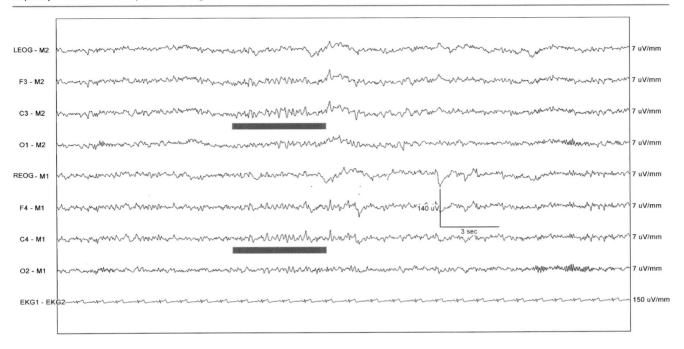

Fig. 1.25 The presence of both irregular, mixed frequency EEG background, and sawtooth waves (*red bars*) in the absence of eye movements makes this a typical epoch of tonic REM

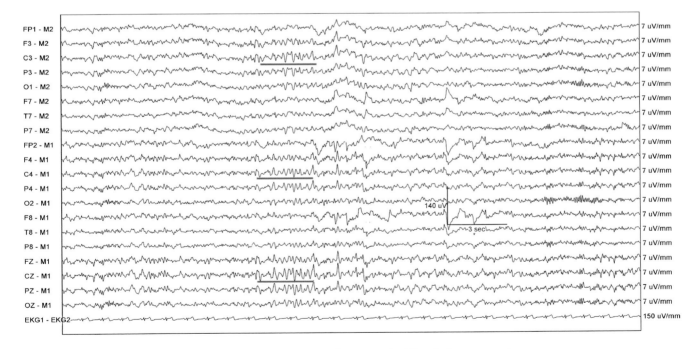

Fig. 1.26 The same epoch as in Fig. 1.25 displaying a full-head EEG montage. *Red lines* indicate sawtooth waves

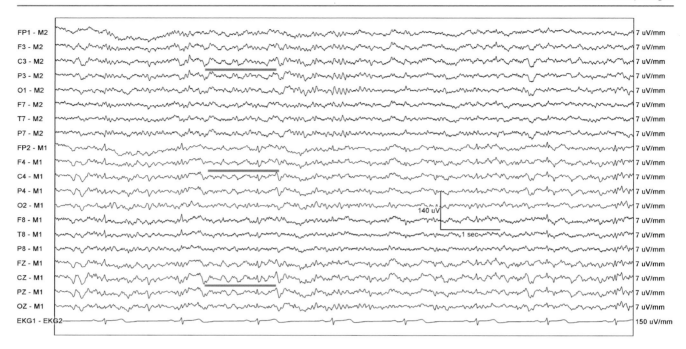

Fig. 1.27 A 10-s portion of the same epoch as in Fig. 1.26 at the faster 30 mm/s paper speed. *Red lines* indicate sawtooth waves

Transition from W to N1

The transition from W to N1 is an important determination, especially when scoring multiple sleep latency tests and maintenance of wakefulness tests. By definition, absence of adequate alpha rhythm is required with a background of 4–7 Hz activity or slowing of the background by ≥1 Hz from that of stage W [3] (Figs. 1.28–1.30).

Arousals

The 2007 *AASM Manual for the Scoring of Sleep and Associated Events* defines arousals as an abrupt shift of EEG frequency (but not spindles) that lasts at least 3 s but not more than 15 s, with at least 10 s of stable sleep preceding the change. In R sleep, an additional concurrent increase in muscle tone is required before an arousal can be scored.

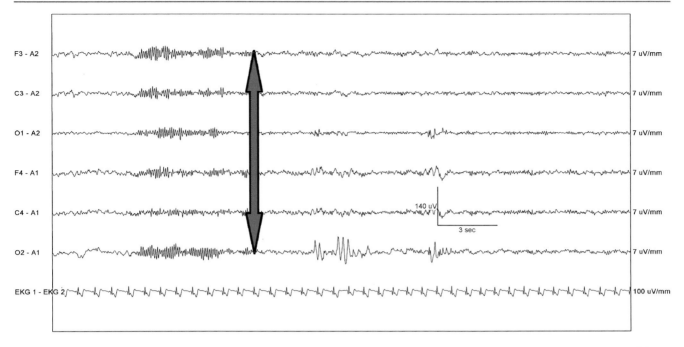

Fig. 1.28 *Bidirectional red arrow* marks the point where stage W gives way to N1. Note the deterioration of alpha rhythms and the onset of slower theta activity

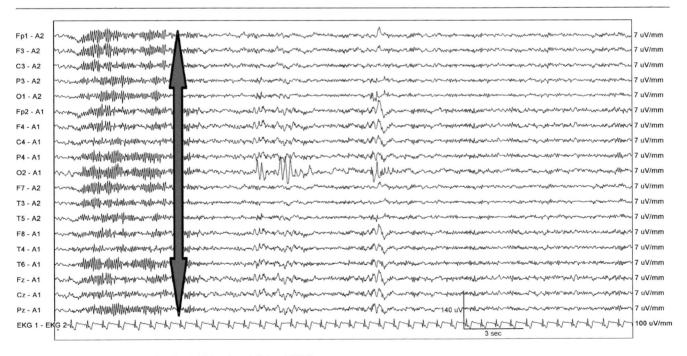

Fig. 1.29 The same epoch as in Fig. 1.28 but in a full-head EEG montage

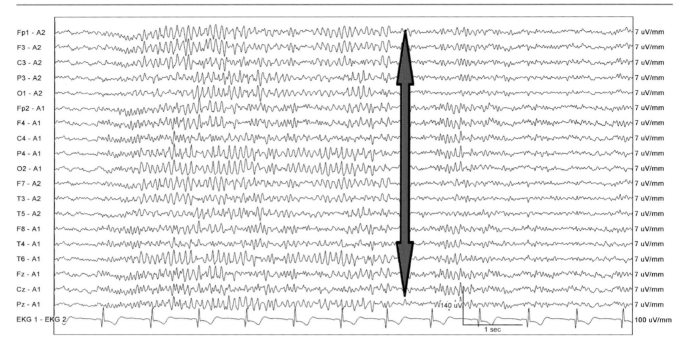

Fig. 1.30 A 10-s window of the epoch in Fig. 1.29 shown in the faster 30 mm/s EEG paper speed

Arousals from N1 (Figs. 1.31–1.33)

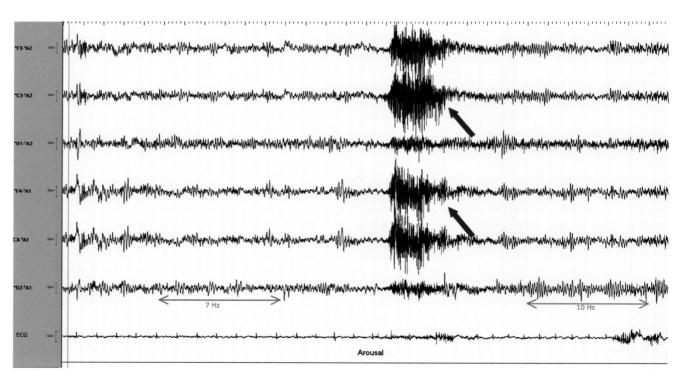

Fig. 1.31 *Red arrows* indicate the shift from 7 Hz to a 10 Hz background. *Blue arrows* point to the arousal and the related EMG artifact

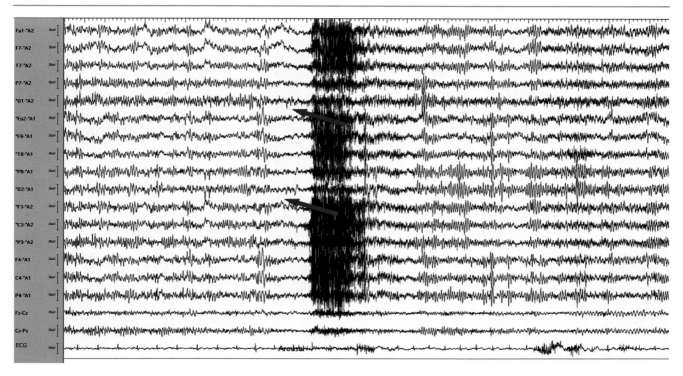

Fig. 1.32 The same epoch as in Fig. 1.31 but with a full EEG montage. *Blue arrows* point to the arousal and the related EMG artifact

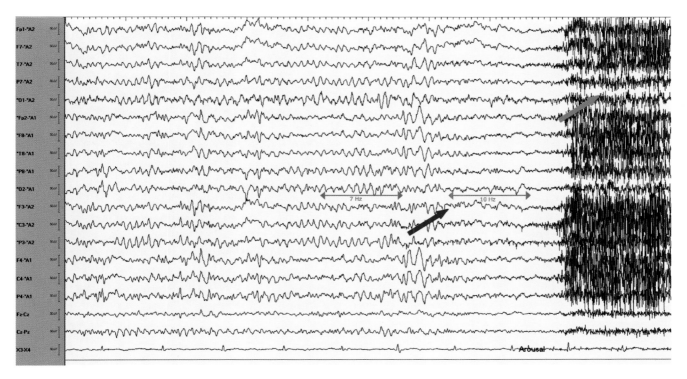

Fig. 1.33 A 10-s window of the same arousal as in Fig. 1.32 but now at the faster EEG paper speed of 30 mm/s. *Red arrows* indicate frequency changes. The *blue arrow* indicates EEG arousal. The *green arrow* indicates the associated EMG artifact. The difference between the two is clearer now with the faster paper speed

Arousals from N2 (Figs. 1.34–1.36)

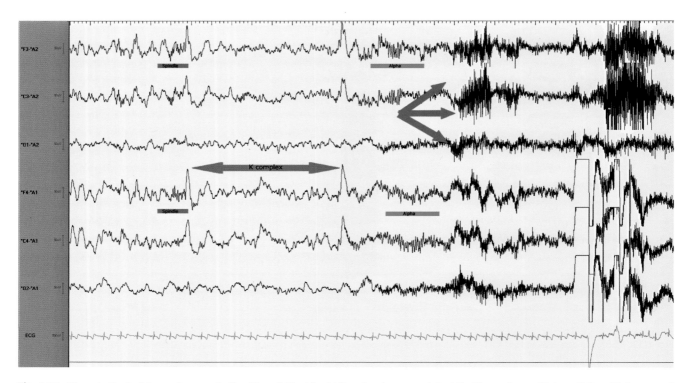

Fig. 1.34 The spindles in this epoch are *underlined in red*. The *blue bidirectional arrow* points at the K complexes. Alpha activity with the arousal is *underlined in green*. The *triple arrow* points to the EMG artifact

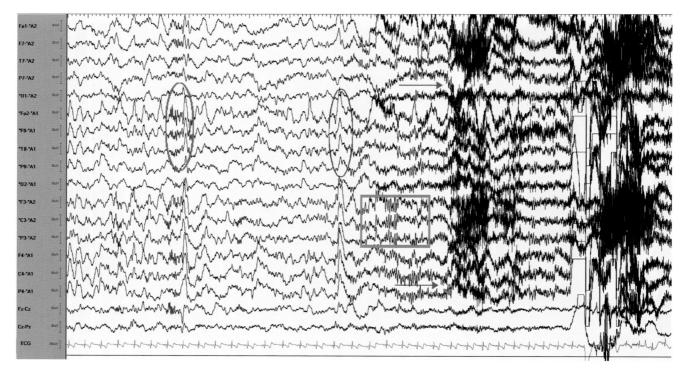

Fig. 1.35 Full-head EEG montage of Fig. 1.34. *Red oval* marks the spindles. *Blue oval* indicates K complexes. The *green square* shows the change in EEG frequency. *Red arrows* indicate the EMG artifact

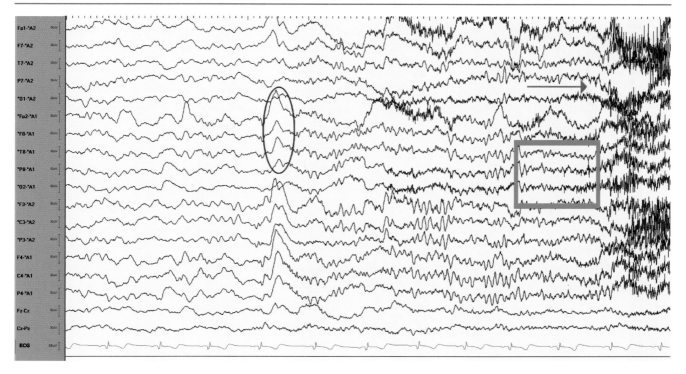

Fig. 1.36 On this 10-s window of Fig. 1.35 at the EEG paper speed, the *blue oval* shows K complexes, the *green square* shows the change in EEG frequency, and the *red arrow* indicates the EMG artifact

N3 Arousals (Figs. 1.37–1.39)

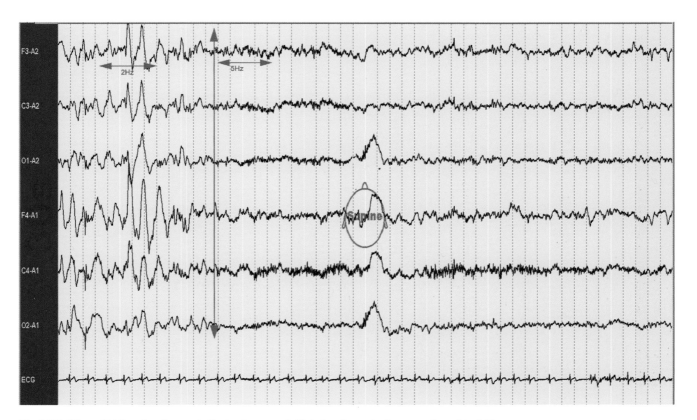

Fig. 1.37 The *red bidirectional arrow* indicates the arousal. Note the change in frequency from 2 to 5 Hz

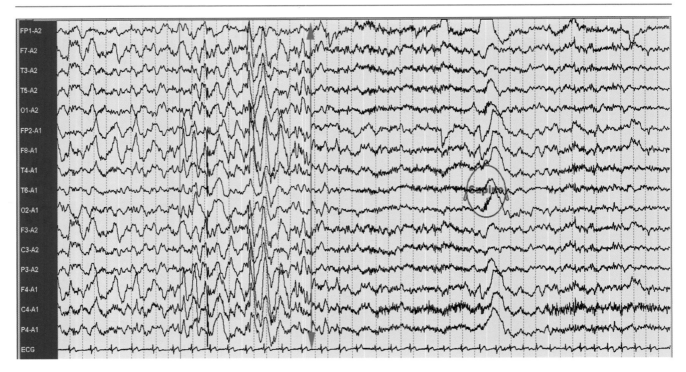

Fig. 1.38 The same epoch as in Fig. 1.37 with the full-head EEG montage. The *red bidirectional arrow* indicates the arousal

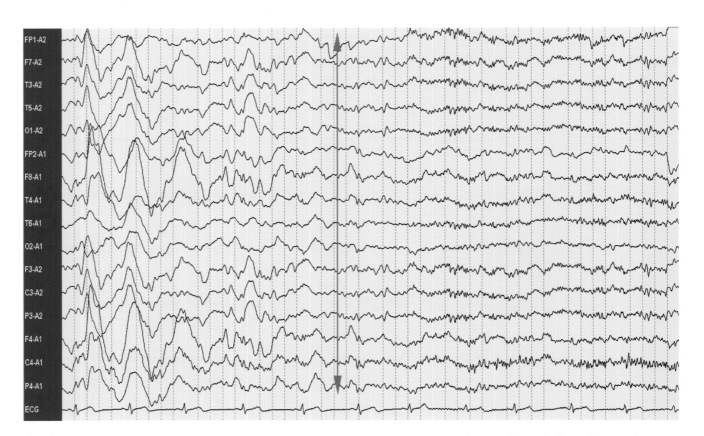

Fig. 1.39 A 10-s window of the same arousal as in Fig. 1.38 at the EEG paper speed. The *red bidirectional arrow* indicates the arousal

R Arousals (Figs. 1.40–1.42)

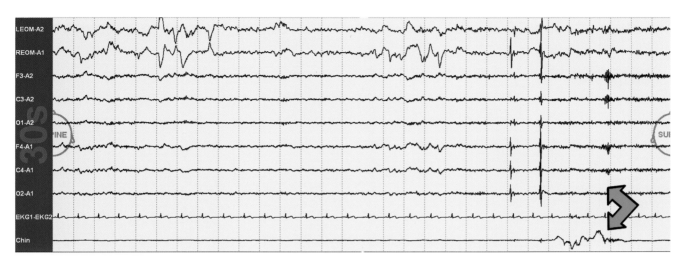

Fig. 1.40 The *two-headed arrow* points at the increase in the EEG frequency and the concomitant increase in the chin EMG tone

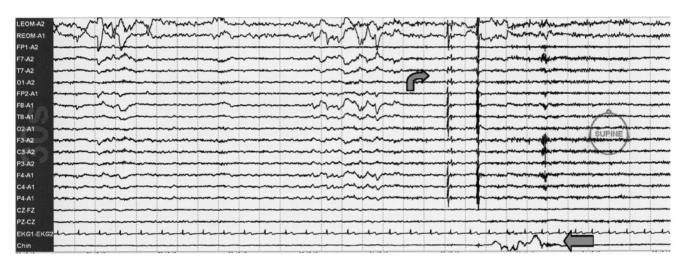

Fig. 1.41 The same epoch as in Fig. 1.40 in a full-head EEG montage. The *curved arrow* points at the EEG portion of the arousal and the *straight arrow* indicates the EMG component

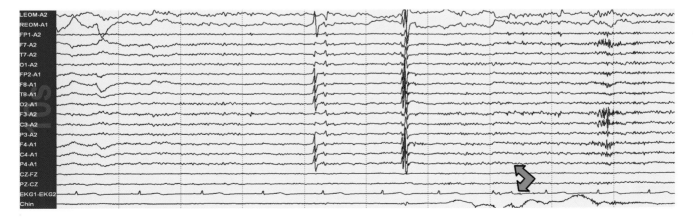

Fig. 1.42 A 10-s window of the same arousal as in Fig. 1.41 at the faster EEG speed. The *two-headed arrow* points at the increase in the EEG frequency and the concomitant increase in the chin EMG tone

References

1. Tatum 4th WO, Husain AM, Benbadis SR, Kaplan PW. Normal adult EEG and patterns of uncertain significance. J Clin Neurophysiol. 2006;23:194–207.
2. Pavlenko VB, Chernyi SV, Goubkina DG. EEG correlates of anxiety and emotional stability in adult healthy subjects. Neurophysiology. 2009;41:337–45.
3. Silber MH, Ancoli-Israel S, Bonnet MH, et al. The visual scoring of sleep in adults. J Clin Sleep Med. 2007;3:121–31.
4. American Academy of Sleep Medicine. The AASM manual for the scoring of sleep and associated events: rules, terminology and technical specifications. Darien, IL: American Academy of Sleep Medicine; 2007.

Normal Electroencephalography Variants in Sleep

2

Keywords

POSTS • Hypnagogic hypersynchrony • Wicket spikes • RMTD • Small sharp spikes • CAP • Breech rhythm

Normal variants, also known as *benign epileptiform variants* (BEVs), are uncommonly occurring waveforms that may appear epileptogenic to the untrained eye. Five BEVs have been described. This chapter shows samples of three BEVs that often occur in sleep and that a sleep specialist may therefore encounter on a polysomnography (PSG). We also show samples of four other electroencephalographic (EEG) phenomena that occur frequently yet may cause confusion in certain situations.

Wicket Spikes

Wicket spikes are BEVs that appear in N1 and N2 sleep, primarily in the frontal and temporal regions. They are rounded on one end and sharp or spiky on the other. Their name derives from their croquet wicket-like shape. They are in theta frequency range, tend to occur exclusively in adults (prevalence, 0.03–0.8%), and are often asymmetrical [1] (Figs. 2.1–2.3).

Rhythmic Midtemporal Theta of Drowsiness

Often confused with wicket spikes, rhythmic midtemporal theta of drowsiness (RMTD) tends to occur exclusively in N1 sleep in adolescents and younger adults (prevalence, 0.5–2%). RMTDs are often asymmetrical and can have a wide electric field but are maximal in the midtemporal electrodes. They last 1–10 s, are higher in amplitude than the wicket, and are sharply contoured, lacking the rounded upswing of the former [1] (Figs. 2.4–2.6).

Small Sharp Spikes

Perhaps the most common of all BEVs (prevalence, 1.4–24%, depending on published series and age groups studied) are the small sharp spikes (SSS) or benign small sharp spikes (BSSS). Formerly known as *benign epileptiform transients of sleep* (BETS), SSSs mostly occur in younger adults. These usually sporadic waveforms occur in N1 and N2 sleep, are often maximal temporally, and tend to be unilateral with a wide electric field [1] (Figs. 2.7–2.9).

Positive Occipital Sharp Transients of Sleep

Positive occipital sharp transients of sleep (POSTS) are a normal phenomenon of primarily N1 and N2 sleep and occur in 8–13% of routine EEGs, but the prevalence increases significantly to 60% if EEGs that contain only wakefulness are excluded. They are asymmetrical in a little more than a third of cases. They are maximal in the occipital areas and tend to be sharp, positive waveforms (downward deflection at the recording electrode) [2] (Figs. 2.10–2.12).

Cyclic Alternating Pattern

Although cyclic alternating pattern (CAP) is associated with some degree of sleep instability, it can be seen in otherwise healthy sleepers and its characteristic pattern shifts may seem abnormal, hence its inclusion in the chapter on normal variants (Figs. 2.13–2.15).

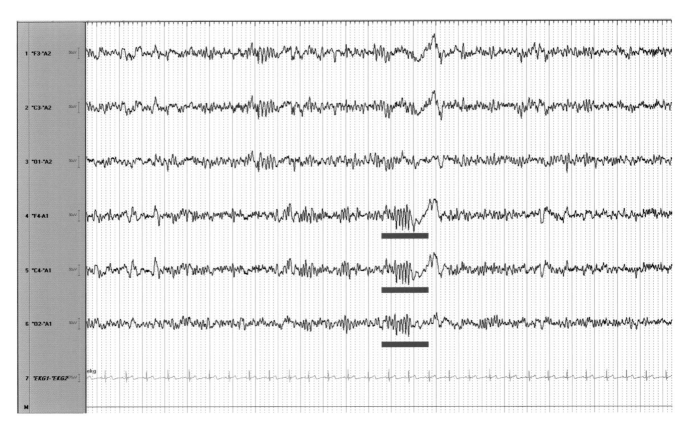

Fig. 2.1 The sample represents N2 sleep. Note the K complexes and the following spindles at 10 mm/s with the PSG montage. Wicket spikes (*underlined in blue*) appear on all right-sided electrodes. They most likely originate over the left temporal lobe and appear in all channels that have input from A1 (left mastoid), an electrode with close proximity to the left temporal area. Note the rounded appearance as it rises and the sharp downward deflection that follows

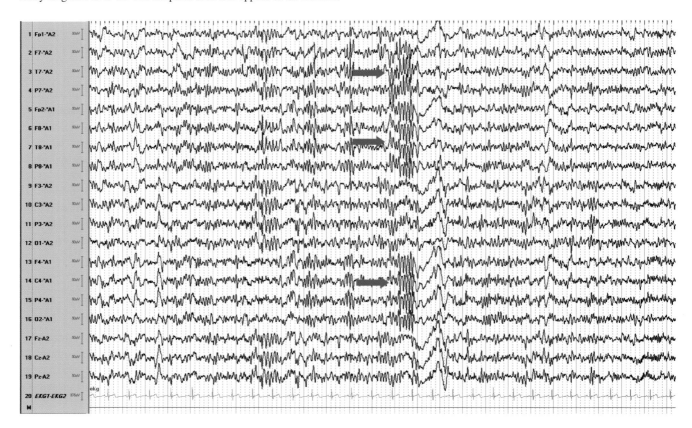

Fig. 2.2 The same 30-s epoch as in Fig. 2.1 but shown in full EEG montage. *Blue arrows* indicate wicket spikes, which are maximal in amplitude at the T7 electrode, confirming the suspicion that they originate in the left temporal area

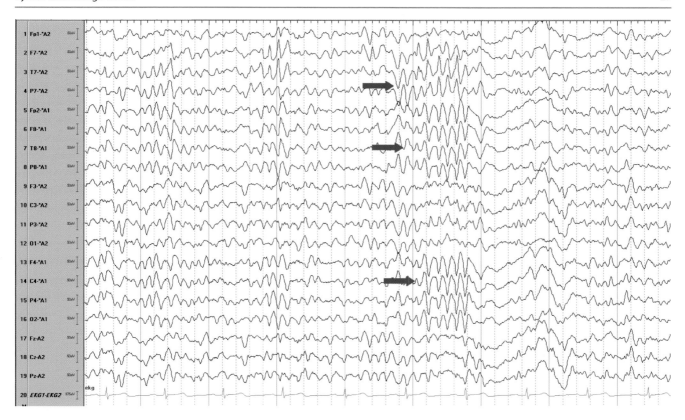

Fig. 2.3 A 10-s sample of the same epoch as in Fig. 2.2 shown at 30 mm/s speed. The wicket-like appearance of the waves (*blue arrows*) is clearer

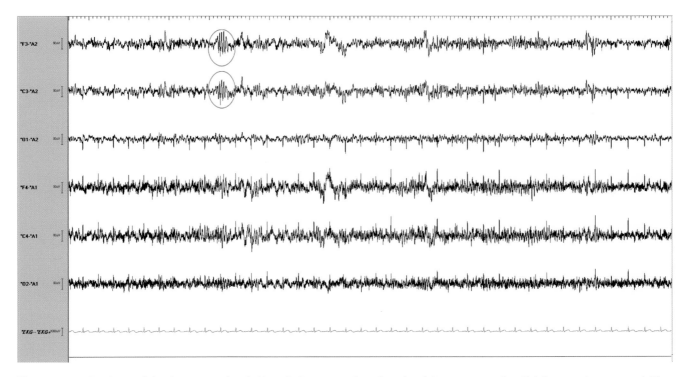

Fig. 2.4 Note the cluster of the sharp waves (*circled in red*) that appear abruptly and end the same way after slightly more than a second. They are maximal at the left frontal and left central electrodes because these are the two closest to the left temporal lobe in this montage

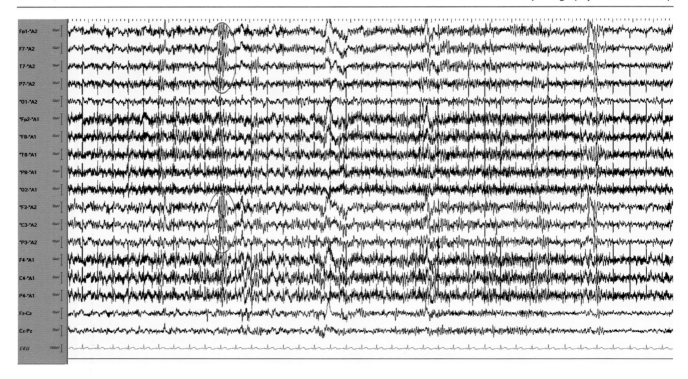

Fig. 2.5 The same epoch as in Fig. 2.4 but with a full EEG montage clearly localizing the RMTD (*circled in red*) to the left temporal electrodes of F7 and T7

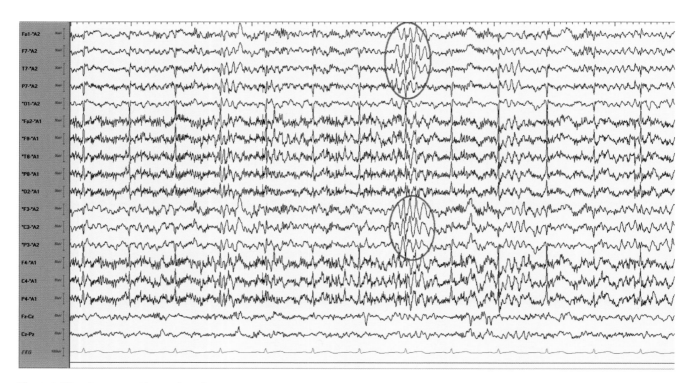

Fig. 2.6 Waveforms on a 10-s portion of the epoch as in Fig. 2.5 at 30 mm/s paper speed. *Red circles* indicate RMTDs. The characteristic mixture of notched and sharply contoured waves is clearer at the faster paper speed

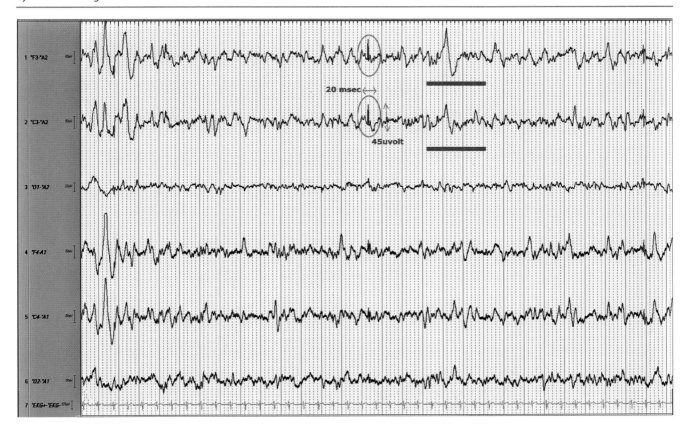

Fig. 2.7 Note the characteristic, extremely steep decline after the first monophasic rise and the small after-going slow wave. As required for an SSS, the duration is shorter than 50 ms (20 ms) and the amplitude is under 50 mV (45 mV). *Blue bars* indicate K complexes, demonstrating that this epoch is N2 sleep

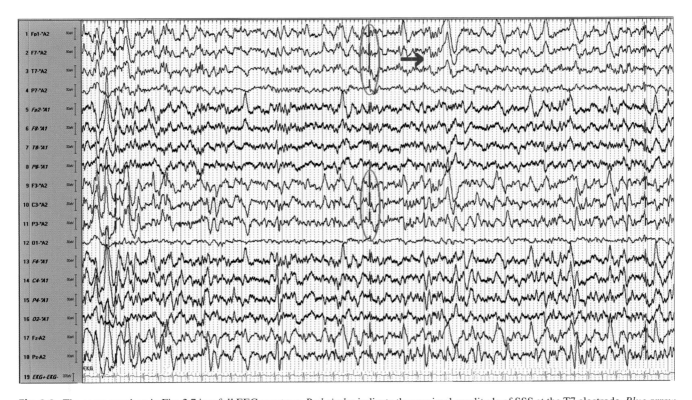

Fig. 2.8 The same epoch as in Fig. 2.7 in a full EEG montage. *Red circles* indicate the maximal amplitude of SSS at the T7 electrode. *Blue arrow* indicates the K complex, demonstrating this is N2 sleep

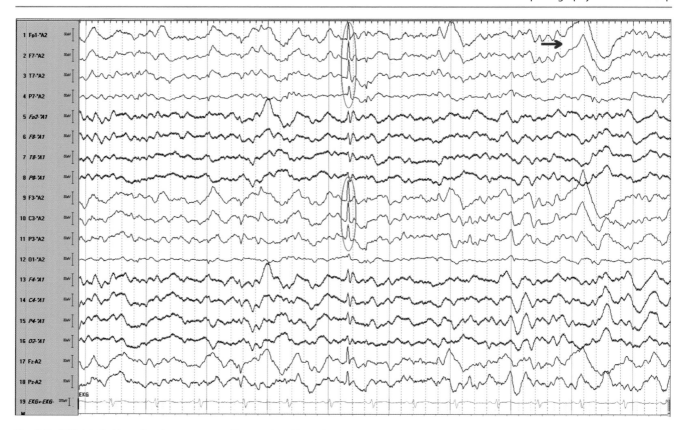

Fig. 2.9 SSS (*circled in red*) as it appears on a 10-s epoch at 30 mm/s paper speed. Its morphology is clearer than in Fig. 2.8. *Blue arrow* indicates the K complex

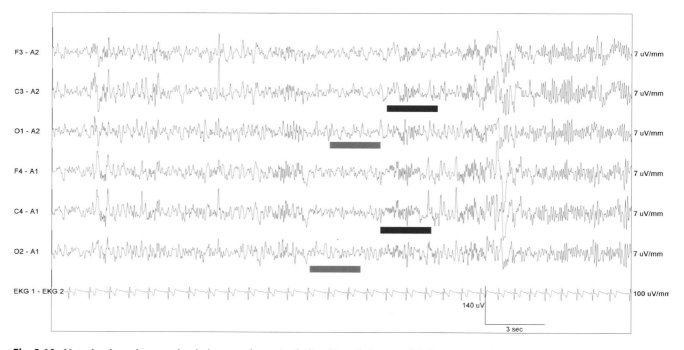

Fig. 2.10 Note the sharp downward-pointing waveforms (*underlined in red*) that are slightly more prominent on the left (O1–A2) than the right (O2–A1). Spindles and K complexes (*underlined in blue*) indicate that the epoch is in N2 sleep

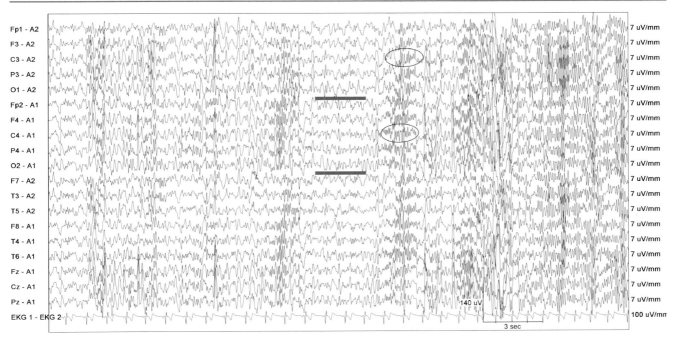

Fig. 2.11 The same epoch as in Fig. 2.10 in a full EEG montage. POSTS (*underlined in red*) are a bit clearer. *Blue circles* indicate spindles

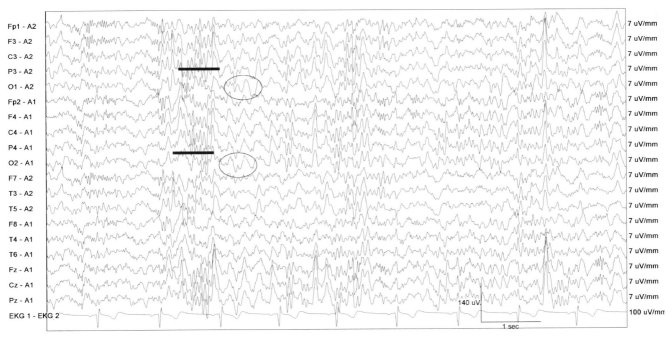

Fig. 2.12 A 10-s epoch at 30 mm/s of the same findings as in Fig. 2.11. The POSTS are clearer (*circled in red*), and the spindles are *underlined in blue*

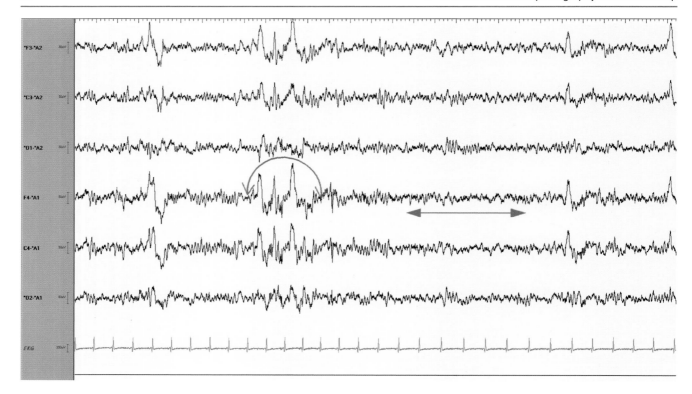

Fig. 2.13 CAP is characterized by two phases: phase A (*curved bidirectional arrow*) consists of transient waveforms that stand out from the background and phase B (*straight bidirectional arrow*), which usually consists of background activity [5]

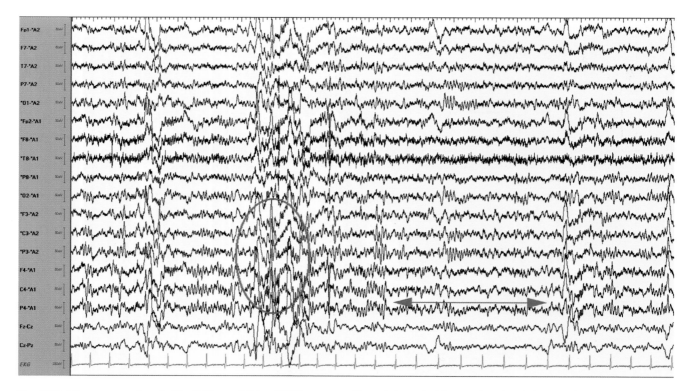

Fig. 2.14 The same epoch as in Fig. 2.13 at a full-head EEG montage. Phase A is marked by a *red oval*, and the *straight bidirectional arrow* indicates phase B

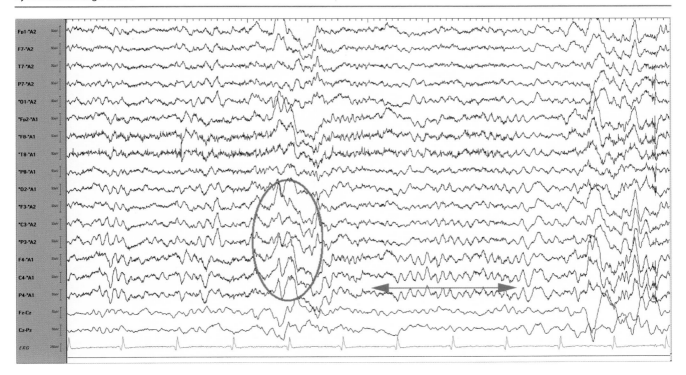

Fig. 2.15 A 10-s portion of the epoch at 30 mm/s paper speed. *Red oval* indicates phase A, and *straight bidirectional arrow* indicates phase B

Breach Rhythm

The human skull acts as a high-frequency filter that blocks any activity higher than 100 Hz from coming through, unless there is a discontinuity in the skull (often postsurgical), in which case focal runs of faster (sometimes mixed with slower waves) and often sharply contoured activity may appear on an EEG channel. This may seem like an epileptiform abnormality because they are often rhythmic but lack of crescendo–decrescendo pattern and absence of slowing afterward are clues to their benign nature (Figs. 2.16–2.18).

Hypnagogic or Hypnopompic Hypersynchrony

Often confused for epileptiform discharges, hypnagogic or hypnopompic hypersynchrony is a paroxysmal, generalized burst of diffuse, synchronous, rhythmic, 3–4.5 Hz, 75–200 mV (often as high as 350 mV) waves that tend to begin abruptly at the beginning (hypnagogic) or end (hypnopompic) of sleep. They tend to start around 3 months of age and become most prominent by 1 year, tending to disappear after adolescence [3]. Very rare cases are described in adulthood, particularly with an underlying sleep disorder that tends to fragment sleep, such as obstructive sleep apnea syndrome (OSAS) or periodic limb movement disorder (PLMD) [4] (Figs. 2.19–2.23).

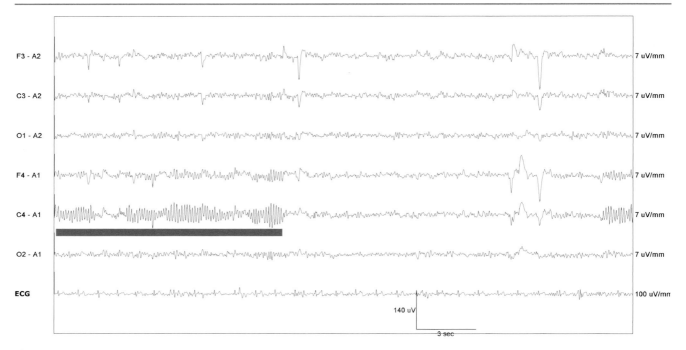

Fig. 2.16 This figure presents the PSG of a 45-year-old man who had undergone right temporal lobectomy. The breach rhythm (*underlined in red*) is best seen in the right central electrode (not an uncommon location) [6, 7]

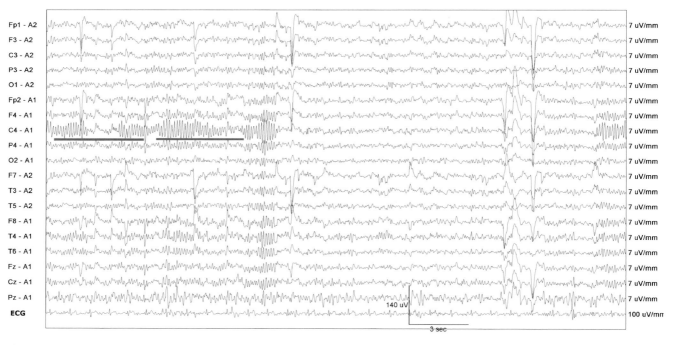

Fig. 2.17 The same epoch as in Fig. 2.16 with a full-head EEG montage. The breach rhythm (*underlined in red*) is best seen in the right central electrode

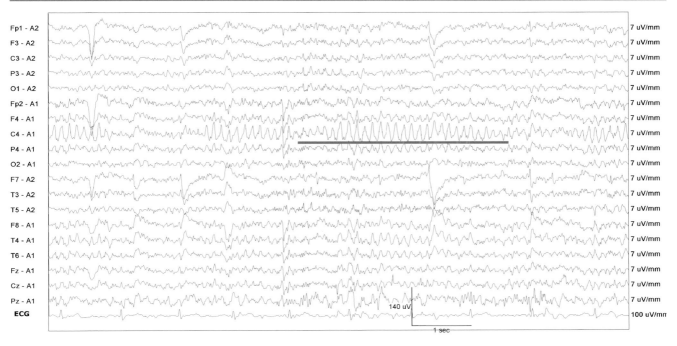

Fig. 2.18 A 10-s portion of the epoch in Fig. 2.17 at 30 mm/s. The benign features of the breach rhythm (*underlined in red*) are clearer at this paper speed

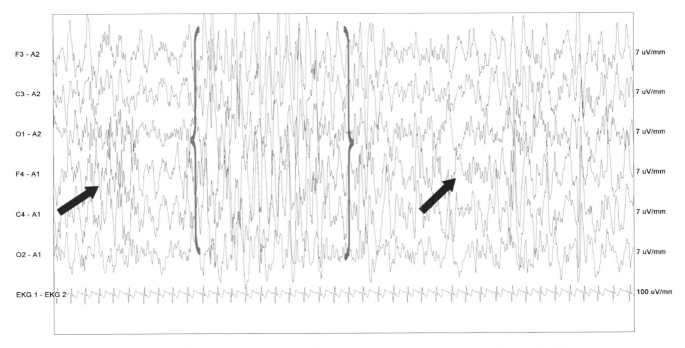

Fig. 2.19 *Blue arrows* indicate spindles, and *red parentheses* indicate hypnopompic hypersynchrony in a 7-year-old child

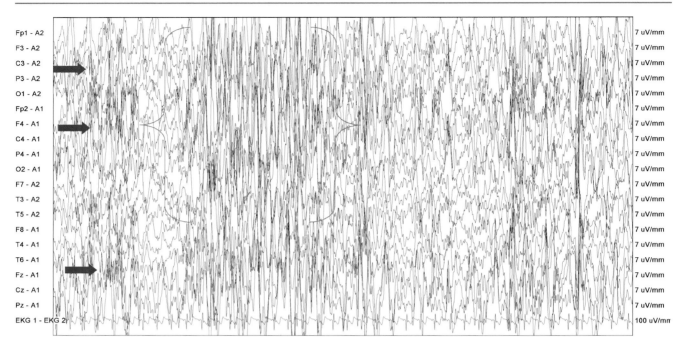

Fig. 2.20 The same epoch as in Fig. 2.19 but with a full-head montage. Because of the extremely high amplitude of the hypersynchrony, a pen limitation effect makes it difficult to see the peak of waves. *Blue arrows* indicate spindles, and the hypersynchrony appears between *red parentheses*

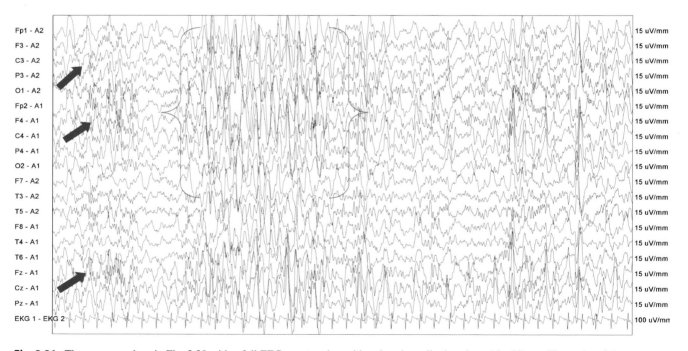

Fig. 2.21 The same epoch as in Fig. 2.20 with a full EEG montage but with reduced amplitude gain at 15 mV/mm. The peaks of the waves are clearly seen now. *Blue arrows* indicate spindles, and hypersynchrony appears between *red parentheses*

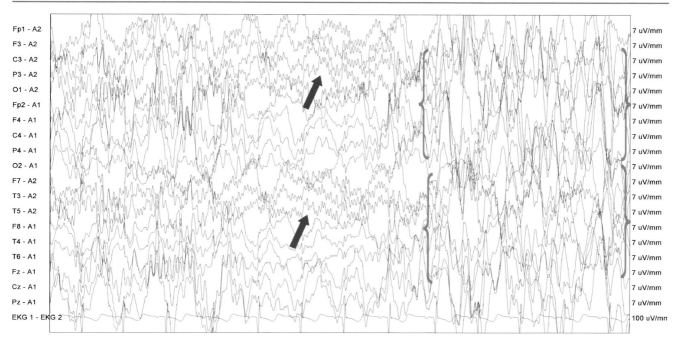

Fig. 2.22 A 10-s portion of the epoch in Fig. 2.21 at 30 mm/s around the hypersynchronous burst. Note the absence of the sharp waves or spikes preceding or mixed in with the rhythmic slow waves. *Blue arrows* indicate spindles, and hypersynchrony appears between *red parentheses*

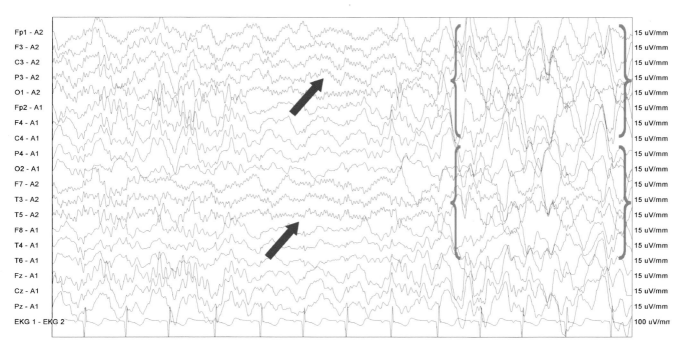

Fig. 2.23 The same epoch as in Fig. 2.22 at the lower amplitude gain of 15 mV/mm, making the absence of sharp waves and spikes clearer. *Blue arrows* indicate spindles, and hypersynchrony appears between *red parentheses*

References

1. Santoshkumar B, Chong JJ, Blume WT, et al. Prevalence of benign epileptiform variants. Clin Neurophysiol. 2009;120:856–61.
2. Rey V, Aybek S, Maeder-Ingvar M, Rossetti AO. Positive occipital sharp transients of sleep (POSTS): a reappraisal. Clin Neurophysiol. 2009;120:472–5.
3. Grigg-Damberger M, Gozal D, Marcus CL, et al. The visual scoring of sleep and arousal in infants and children. J Clin Sleep Med. 2007;3:201–40.
4. Tatum WO, Spector A. Physiologic pseudoseizures: an EEG case report of mistake in identity. J Clin Neurophysiol. 2011;28: 308–10.
5. Parrino L, Ferri R, Bruni O, Terzano MG. Cyclic alternating pattern (CAP): the marker of sleep instability. Sleep Med Rev. 2012;16(1): 27–45.
6. Westmoreland BF, Klass DW. Unusual EEG patterns. J Clin Neurophysiol. 1990;7:209–28.
7. Cobb WA, Guiloff RJ, Cast J. Breach rhythm: the EEG related to skull defects. Electroencephalogr Clin Neurophysiol. 1979;47: 251–71.

Nonepileptiform Abnormalities

Keywords

Triphasic waves • FIRDA • Paradoxical arousal • Hemispheric asymmetry (spindle asymmetry)

This chapter covers four abnormal electroencephalogram (EEG) patterns that occur in patients with underlying neurological dysfunction whose condition is stable enough to allow them to visit a sleep center for polysomnographic (PSG) evaluation.

Triphasic Waves

Triphasic waves were first described in liver failure. Although still best seen in patients with hepatic disease, they can occur in a variety of toxic metabolic encephalopathies and rarely may appear on PSGs. As the term *triphasic* indicates, these waves have three phases: (1) a small positive phase, which sometimes is blunted; (2) a large negative phase; and (3) a large positive phase. They also have a characteristic antero-posterior lag and tend to be centrally prominent. In sleep, they tend to be more prominent in stage N1 and after arousal [1] (Figs. 3.1–3.3).

Frontal Intermittent Rhythmic Delta Activity

Frontal intermittent rhythmic delta activity (FIRDA) is characterized by rhythmic bursts of slow frontal waveforms. They are usually seen in the setting of underlying structural abnormalities that range from hydrocephalus to stroke and even basilar migraine. They are seen in wakefulness and disappear with sleep. This PSG is from a 70-year-old man with diffuse ischemic white matter disease [2] (Figs. 3.4–3.6).

Paradoxical Arousal

As discussed in Chap. 1, arousals are usually characterized by faster frequencies than those dominating the sleep stage in which they occur. Occasionally, patterns known as *paradoxical arousals* are seen on PSGs. These are characterized by high amplitude bursts of delta frequency slowing and, although more frequently encountered during recovery from anesthesia, they can occur in the setting of obstructive sleep apnea [3, 4] (Figs. 3.7–3.9).

Spindle Asymmetry

Spindles are generated from thalamocortical projections and, therefore, are most often symmetrical and synchronous. In the setting of structural lesions or even epilepsy, however, there may be an asymmetry of spindle formation and activity. Below is the case of a 60-year-old man with a right thalamic infarct [5] (Figs. 3.10–3.12).

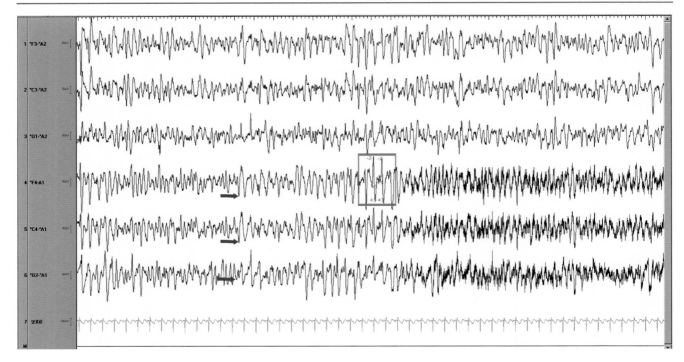

Fig. 3.1 This epoch was scored as N1 and demonstrates triphasic waves throughout. The three phases of the waves (*red rectangle*) are numbered and their polarity is indicated by a positive (+) or negative (−) sign. (Positive is downward by convention and negative is upward.) *Blue arrows* indicate the few millisecond lag of phase one as the waves propagate from frontal to occipital derivations

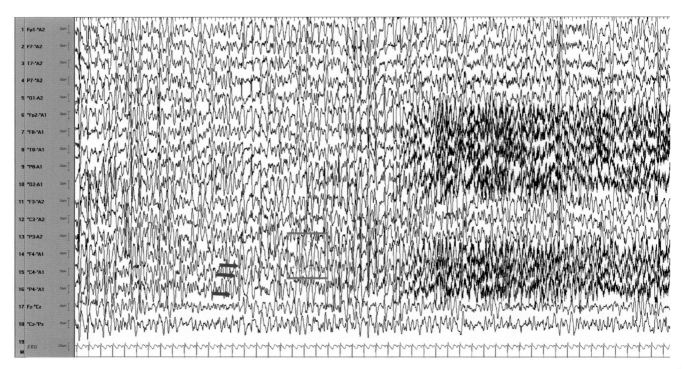

Fig. 3.2 The same epoch as in Fig. 3.1 in a full-head EEG montage. The three phases of the waves (*red rectangle*) are numbered and their polarity is indicated by a positive (+) or negative (−) sign. (Positive is downward by convention and negative is upward.) The anteroposterior lag is clearer here (*blue arrows*)

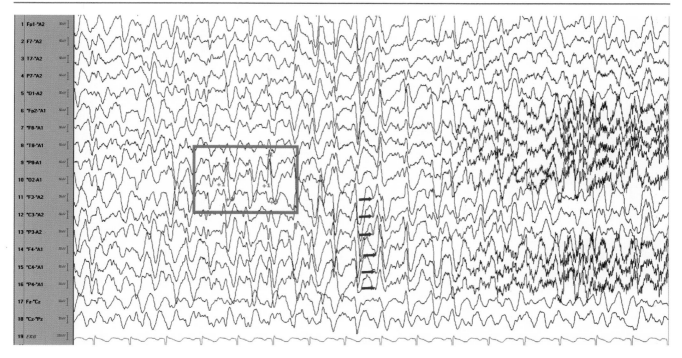

Fig. 3.3 A 10-s portion of the same epoch as in Fig. 3.2 at 30 mm/s paper speed. The three phases of the waves (*red rectangle*) are numbered and their polarity is indicated by a positive (+) or negative (−) sign. The anteroposterior lag is clearer here (*blue arrows*) as is the central prominence of the waves

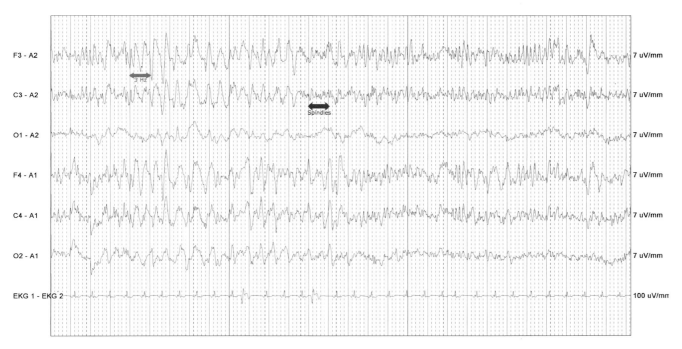

Fig. 3.4 *Red double arrow* indicates the 3-Hz frontal activity that is somewhat rhythmic and disappears when the patient is in stage N2 sleep (*blue double arrow* indicates spindles). Most likely because of extensive ischemia, this patient is unable to generate good alpha activity in the occipital channels

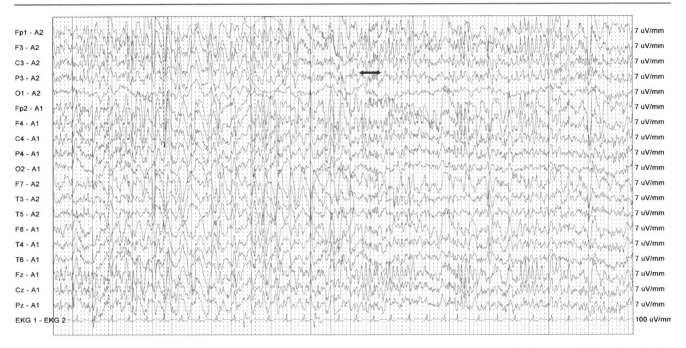

Fig. 3.5 The same epoch as in Fig. 3.4 but with a full-head EEG montage. *Red circles* indicate FIRDA. *Blue double arrow* indicates the spindle

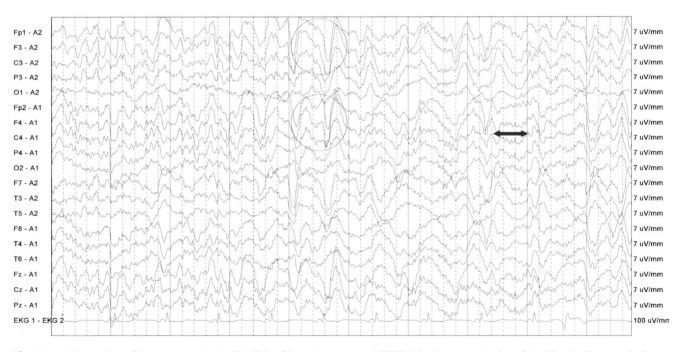

Fig. 3.6 A 10-s portion of the same epoch as in Fig. 3.5 at 30 mm/s paper speed. FIRDA is clearer now (*red circles*). *Blue double arrow* indicates the spindle

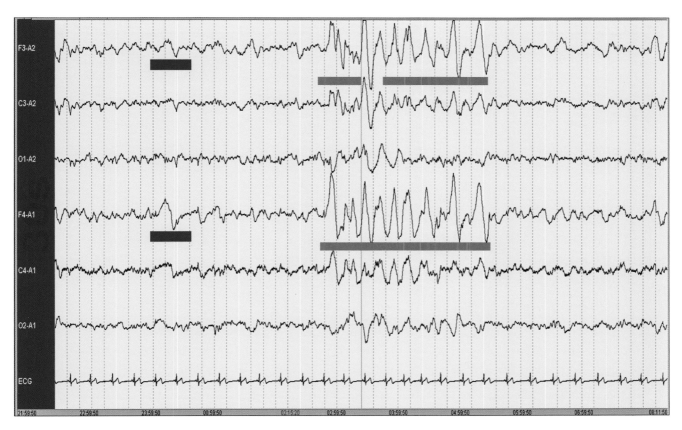

Fig. 3.7 Paradoxical arousal in a PSG. *Red bars* underline arousal characterized by frontally predominant, slow waves. *Blue bars* underline K complexes, indicating stage N2 sleep

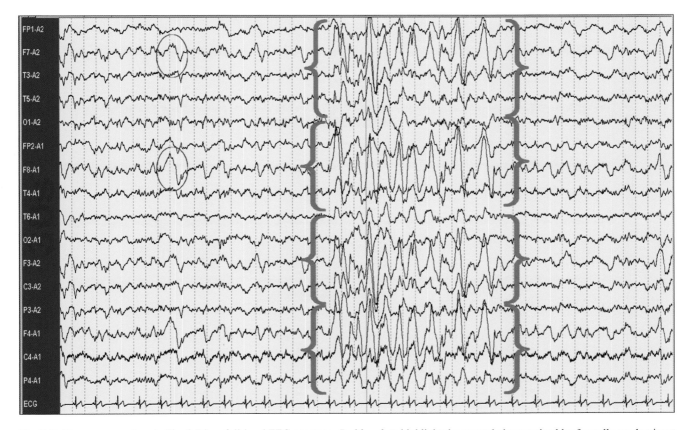

Fig. 3.8 The same epoch as in Fig. 3.7 in a full-head EEG montage. *Red brackets* highlight the arousal characterized by frontally predominant slow waves. *Blue circles* show K complexes, indicating stage N2 sleep

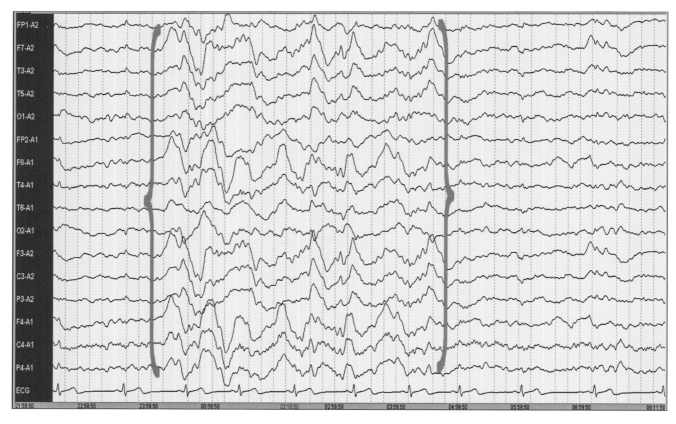

Fig. 3.9 A 10-s portion of the above epoch as in Fig. 3.8 at 30 mm/s. Arousal is characterized by frontally predominant, large amplitude, delta frequency waves (*red brackets*)

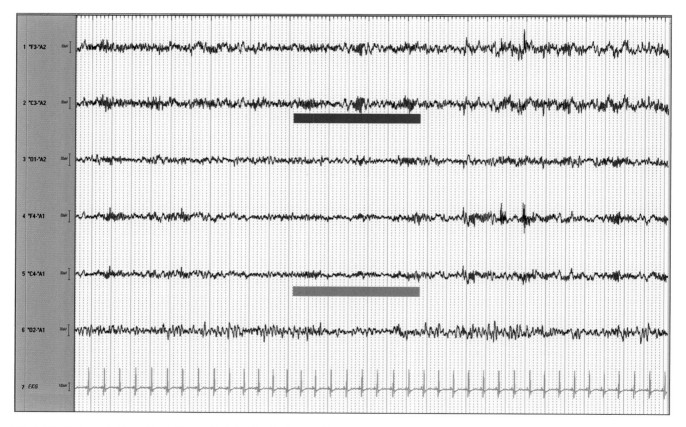

Fig. 3.10 Note nicely formed spindles on the left (*blue bar*) and their absence (*red bar*)

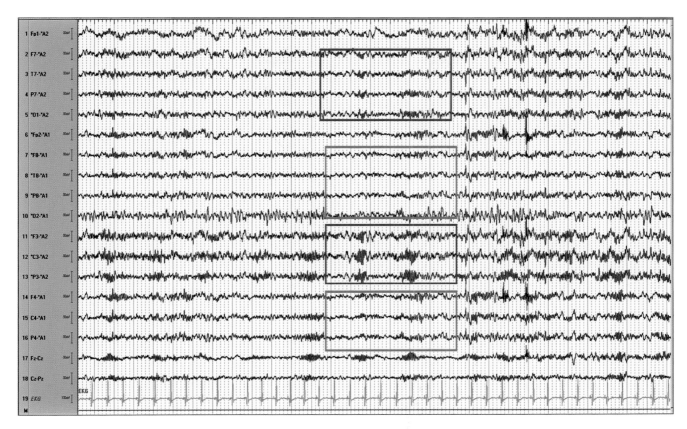

Fig. 3.11 The same epoch as in Fig. 3.10 with a full-head EEG montage. Channels with well-formed spindles (*blue rectangles*) are highlighted on the left and the corresponding channels without spindles (*red rectangles*) are on the right. Also note overall slower rhythms within those channels on the right compared to those on the left

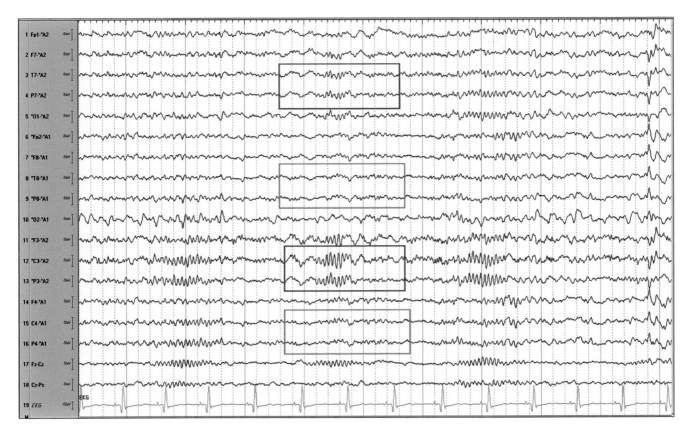

Fig. 3.12 A 10-s portion of the same epoch as in Fig. 3.11 at the usual EEG paper speed of 30 mm/s. The channels with well-formed spindles (*blue rectangles*) are on the left and the corresponding channels without spindles (*red rectangles*) are on the right. The overall right-sided slowing is clearer in this view

References

1. Kaplan PW, Rossetti AO. EEG patterns and imaging correlations in encephalopathy: encephalopathy part II. J Clin Neurophysiol. 2011;28:233–51.
2. Accolla EA, Kaplan PW, Maeder-Ingvar M, et al. Clinical correlates of frontal intermittent rhythmic delta activity (FIRDA). Clin Neurophysiol. 2011;122:27–31.
3. MacKay EC, Sleigh JW, Voss LJ, Barnard JP. Episodic waveforms in the electroencephalogram during general anaesthesia: a study of patterns of response to noxious stimuli. Anaesth Intensive Care. 2010;38:102–12.
4. Tatum WO, Spector A. Physiologic pseudoseizures: an EEG case report of mistake in identity. J Clin Neurophysiol. 2011;28:308–10.
5. Clemens B, Ménes A. Sleep spindle asymmetry in epileptic patients. Clin Neurophysiol. 2000;111:2155–9.

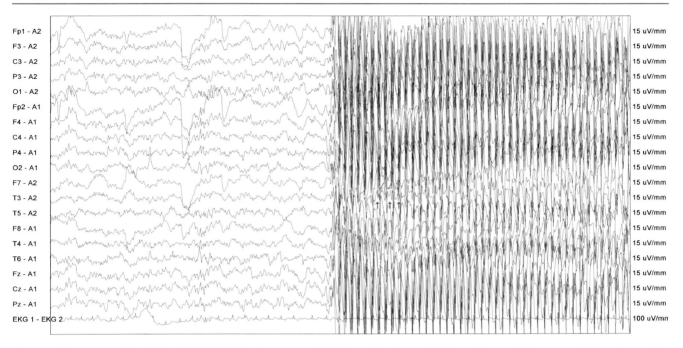

Fig. 4.7 The same epoch as in Fig. 4.6 with full-head montage at 15 mV/mm. *Red arrows* indicate spikes and *blue arrows* indicate the ensuing slow waves

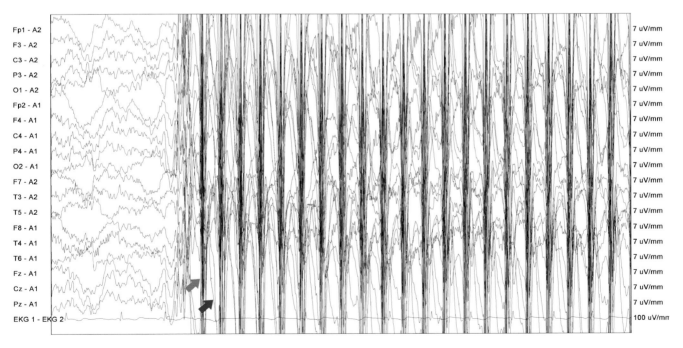

Fig. 4.8 A 10-s portion of Fig. 4.6 at the faster 30 mm/s speed. *Red arrow* indicates the spike and *blue arrow* indicates the ensuing slow wave

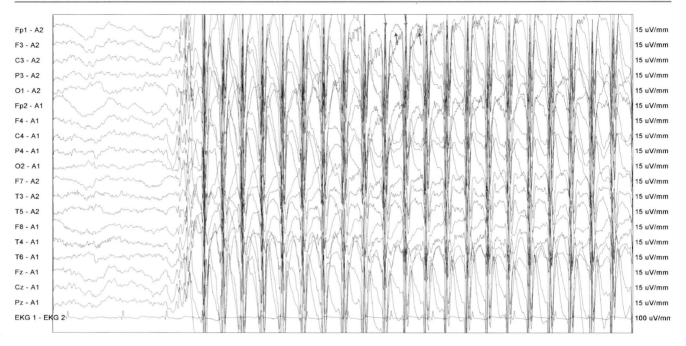

Fig. 4.9 The same epoch as Fig. 4.8 with a lower gain of 15 mV/mm. The frontal predominance is clearer at the reduced gain. *Red arrows* indicate the spikes and *blue arrows* indicate ensuing slow waves. The 30 mm/s paper speed makes the frequency of 3 Hz easier to appreciate

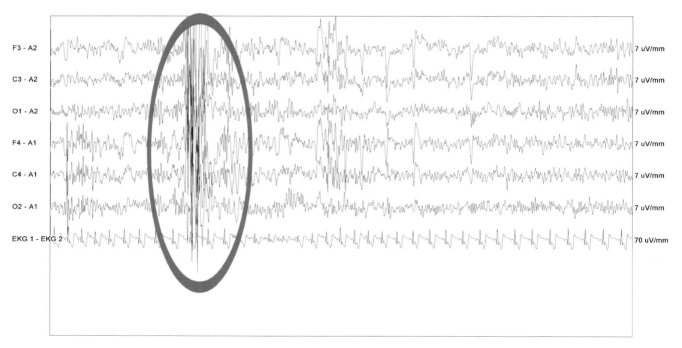

Fig. 4.10 *Red oval* indicates a burst of generalized, fast polyspike, slow-wave activity. Note multiple spikes overriding slow components

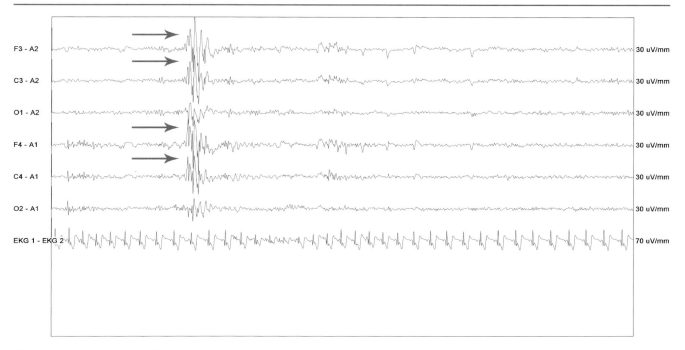

Fig. 4.11 The same epoch as Fig. 4.10 with the gain turned down to 30 mV/mm to clarify the polyspikes (*red arrows*)

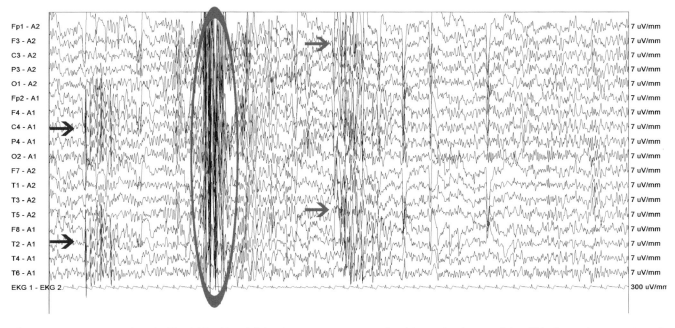

Fig. 4.12 The same epoch as in Fig. 4.10 with a full-head montage. *Red oval* indicates a burst of the generalized, fast polyspike, slow-wave activity. *Red arrows* indicate the left predominant activity and *blue arrows* the right predominant activity. This fluctuating asymmetry is typical of this pattern

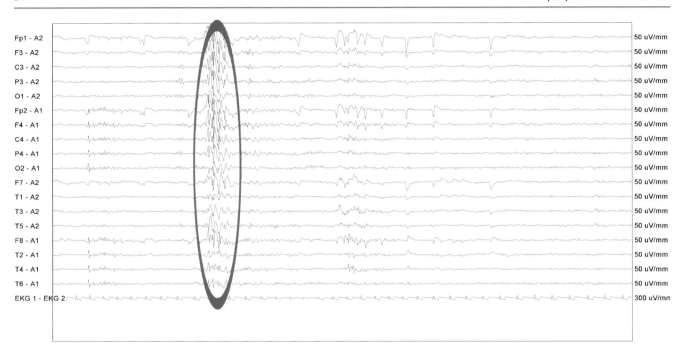

Fig. 4.13 The same epoch as in Fig. 4.12 with the gain turned down to 50 mV/mm to clarify the polyspikes (*red oval*)

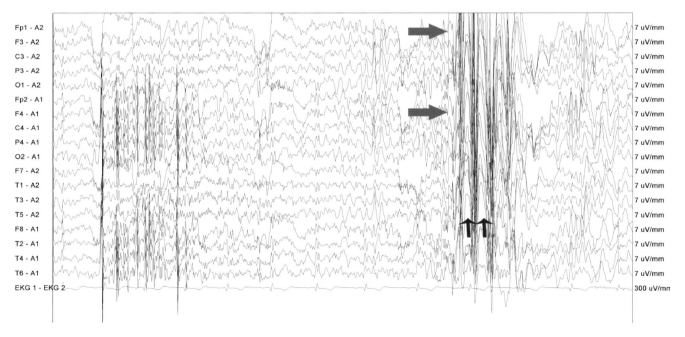

Fig. 4.14 A 10-s portion of Fig. 4.12 at the faster 30 mm/s speed. *Red arrows* indicate the spike and *blue arrows* indicate the ensuing slow wave

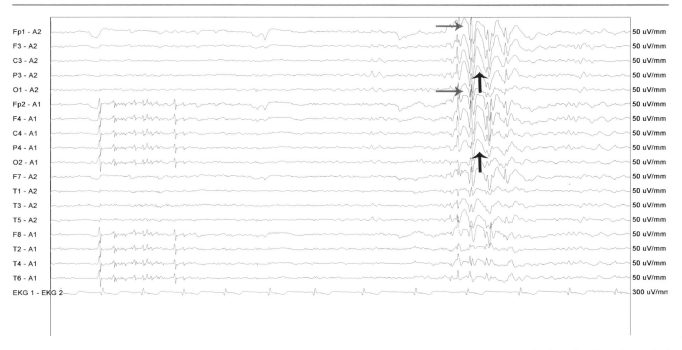

Fig. 4.15 A 10-s portion of Fig. 4.14 at the faster 30 mm/s speed. The gain is turned down to 50 mV/mm to make the polyspikes clearer. *Red arrows* indicate the polyspikes and *blue arrows* indicate the ensuing slow waves

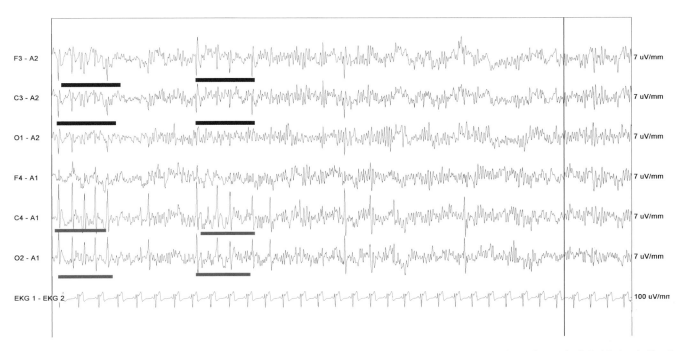

Fig. 4.16 Discharges (*underlined in red*) appear over the right frontal and central electrodes, as well as on electrodes on the left side (*underlined in blue*), because these electrodes reference the A2, which is very close to the right temporal lobe

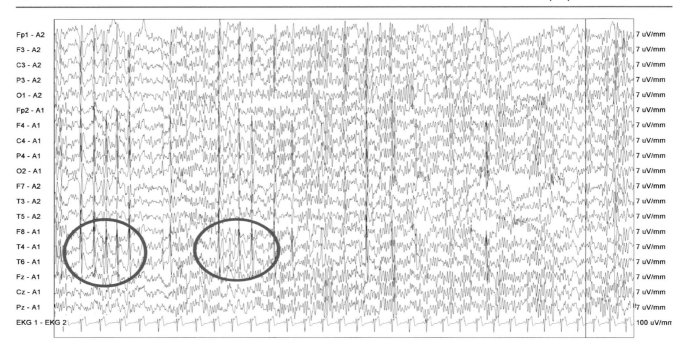

Fig. 4.17 The same epoch as in Fig. 4.16 with a full-head montage. It is clearer now that the discharges (*circled in red*) are primarily in the right anterior and mid-temporal electrodes (F8–T6)

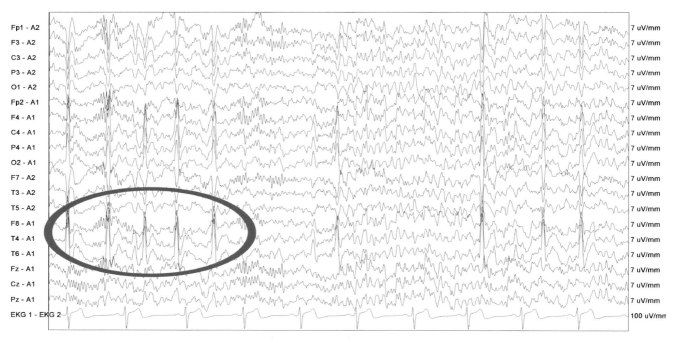

Fig. 4.18 A 10-s portion of Fig. 4.17 at the faster 30 mm/s speed. It is clearer now that the sharp wave discharges (*circled in red*) are primarily in the right anterior and mid-temporal electrodes (F8–T6)

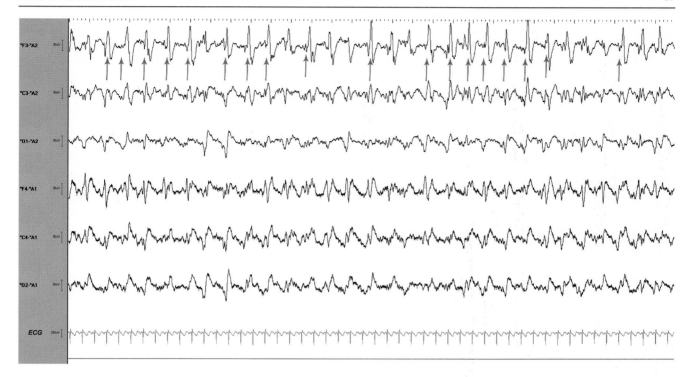

Fig. 4.19 PLEDs (*red arrows*) in the left frontal region as seen on the limited PSG montage

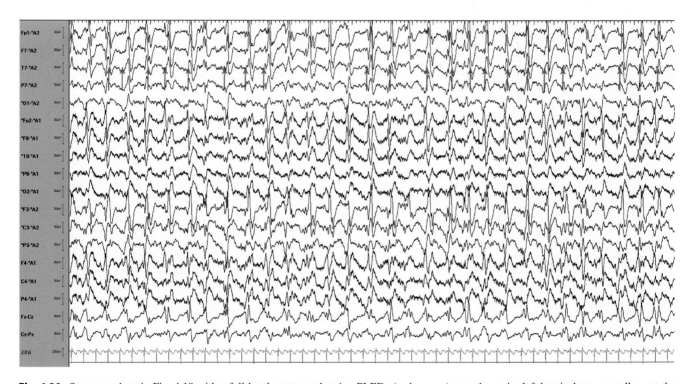

Fig. 4.20 Same epoch as in Fig. 4.19 with a full-head montage showing PLEDs (*red arrows*) over the entire left hemisphere, as well as on the right side (inverted positive waveforms), because the A1 reference electrode captures them due to its proximity to the left temporal lobe

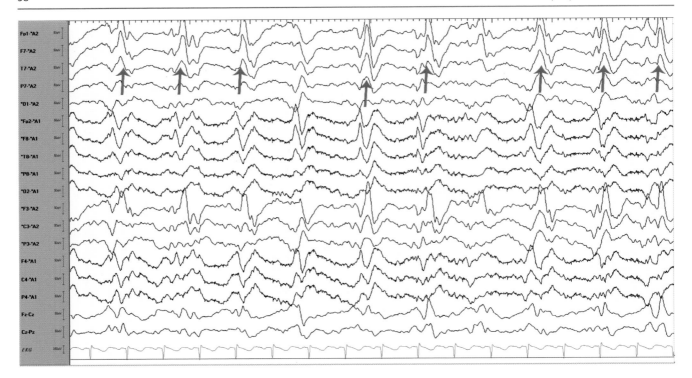

Fig. 4.21 A 10-s portion of Fig. 4.20 at the faster 30 mm/s speed showing PLEDs (*red arrows*) over the entire left hemisphere and showing on the right side are the inverted positive waveforms captured at the A1 reference electrode because of its proximity to the left temporal lobe

desynchrony; lower-voltage fast activity; or irregular focal, rarely bilateral, slow activity. The evolution of the seizure usually involves very distinct progress from lower amplitude with faster activity to higher amplitude activity with slower frequencies. As the seizure ends, the discharges merge into slow activity that is distinctly less rhythmic than the ictal discharge [4] (Figs. 4.22–4.35).

Generalized Seizures

The electrographic hallmark of generalized seizure discharge is the abrupt, bilateral, and synchronous onset over all areas of the cerebrum [2] (Figs. 4.36–4.38).

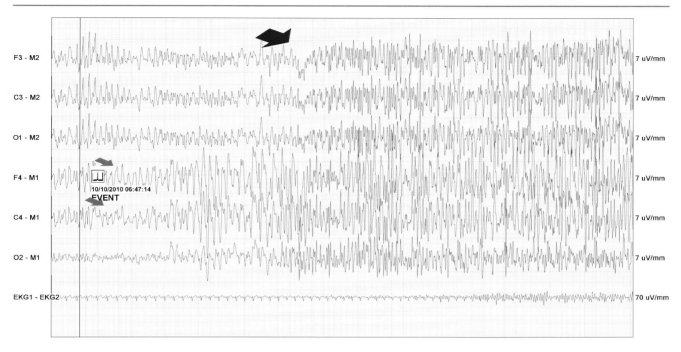

Fig. 4.22 *Red arrows* indicate the start of the seizure. Note the lower voltage, faster activity starting at the F4 and C4 channels followed by higher amplitude, more rhythmic, and generalized slower activities as it evolves here (*blue arrow*)

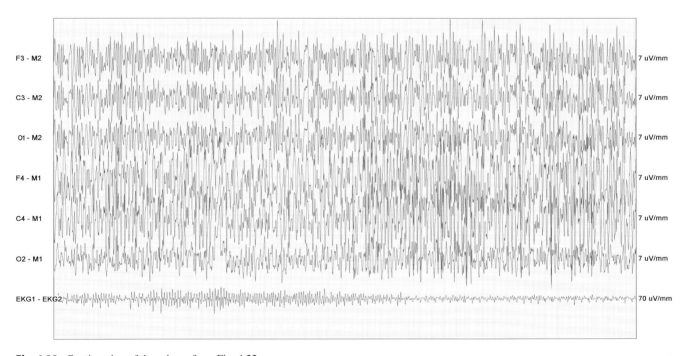

Fig. 4.23 Continuation of the seizure from Fig. 4.22

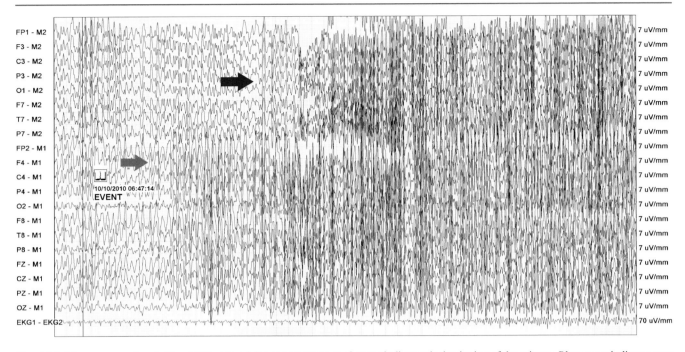

Fig. 4.24 The same epoch as in Fig. 4.22 but in a full-head montage. *Red arrow* indicates the beginning of the seizure. *Blue arrow* indicates start of the evolution

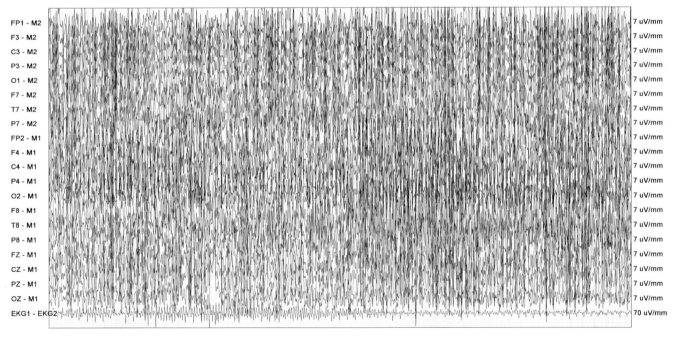

Fig. 4.25 Continuation of the seizure from Fig. 4.24 in a full-head montage

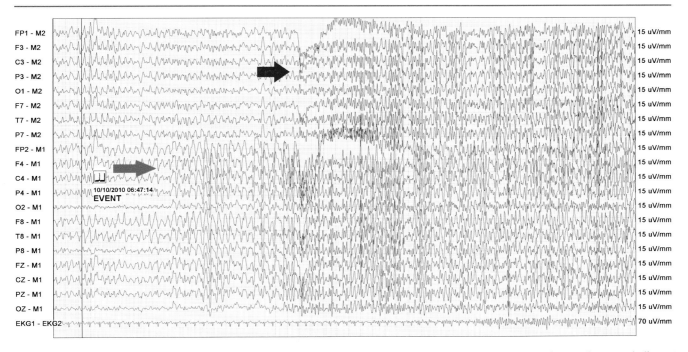

Fig. 4.26 The same epoch as in Fig. 4.24 but at lower gain of 15 mV/mm. *Red arrow* indicates the beginning of the seizure. *Blue arrow* indicates start of the evolution

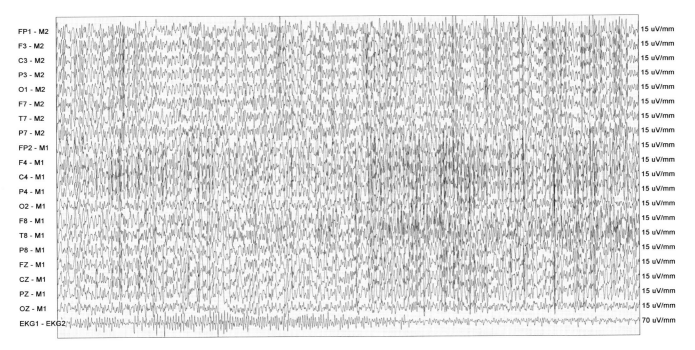

Fig. 4.27 Continuation of the seizure from Fig. 4.26 at lower gain of 15 mV/mm

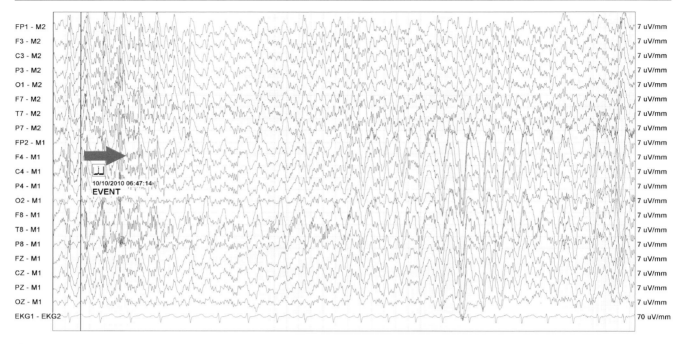

Fig. 4.28   A portion of Fig. 4.24 at the faster 30 mm/s paper speed. *Red arrow* indicates the onset of the seizure

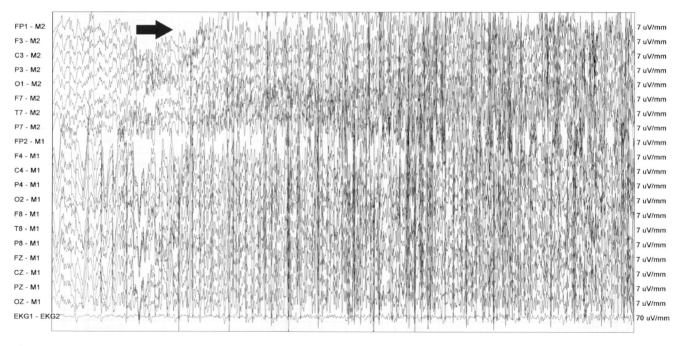

Fig. 4.29   Another portion of Fig. 4.24 at the faster 30 mm/s paper speed. *Blue arrow* indicates the beginning of the evolution and the generalization

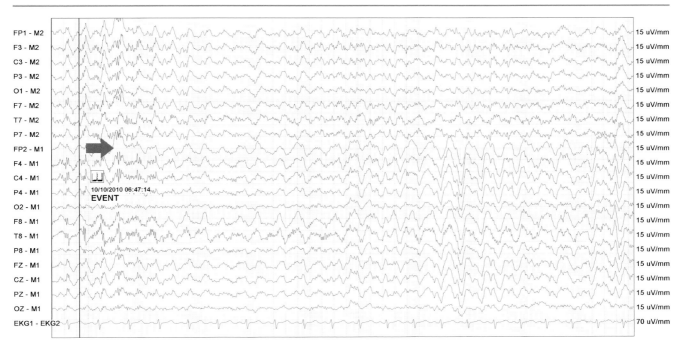

Fig. 4.30 The same epoch in Fig. 4.28 but at the lower gain of 15 mV/mm. *Red arrow* indicates the onset of the seizure

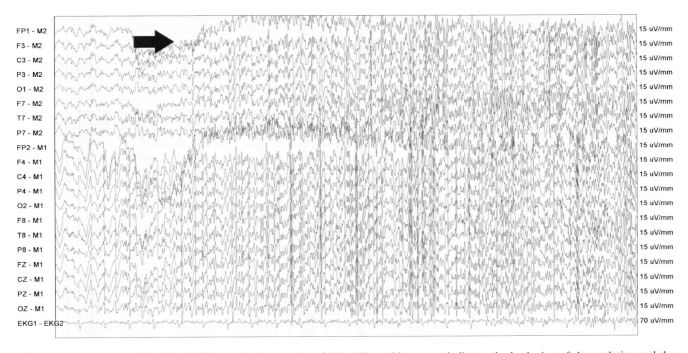

Fig. 4.31 The same epoch in Fig. 4.29 but at the lower gain of 15 mV/mm. *Blue arrow* indicates the beginning of the evolution and the generalization

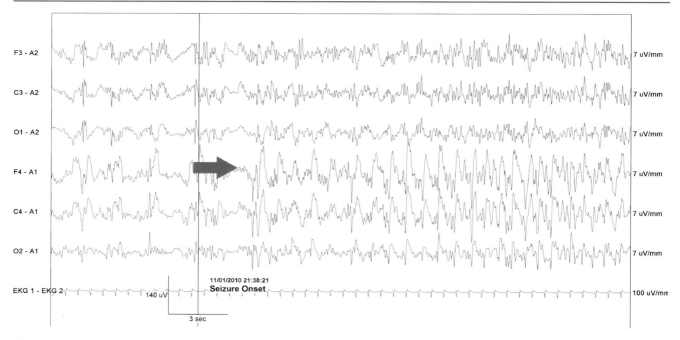

Fig. 4.32 Another focal seizure without generalization. *Red arrow* indicates the point of evolution. Note the desynchrony and the suppression preceding it on the F4 and C4 channels

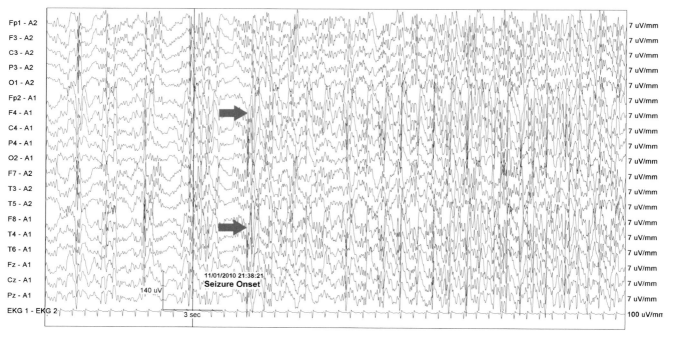

Fig. 4.33 The same epoch as in Fig. 4.32 but in a full-head montage. *Red arrows* indicate the point of evolution

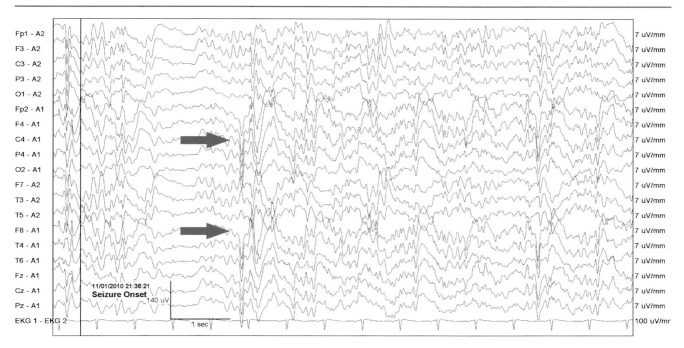

Fig. 4.34 A portion of Fig. 4.33 at the faster 30 mm/s paper speed. *Red arrows* indicate the point of the evolution of the seizure. The presence of the pre-evolution suppression is now clearer

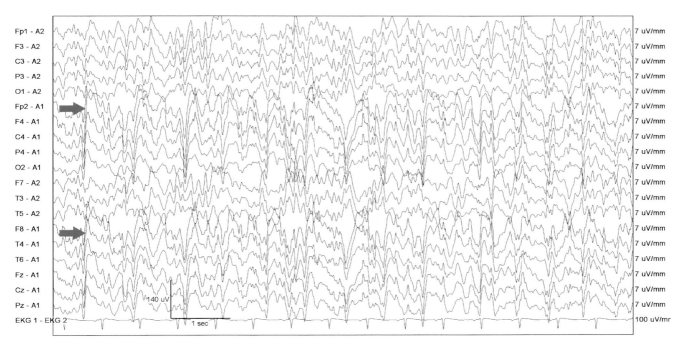

Fig. 4.35 *Red arrows* indicate continuation of seizure activity from Fig. 4.34

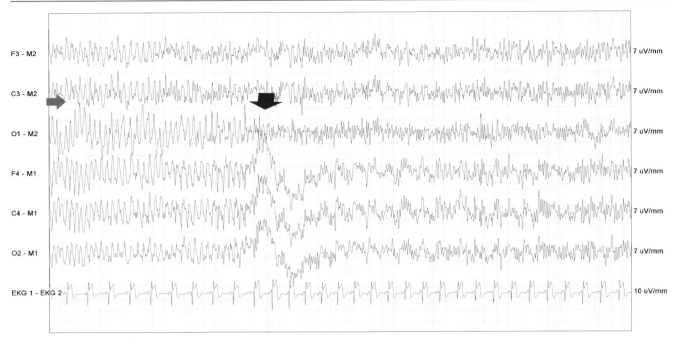

Fig. 4.36 Generalized seizure. *Red arrow* indicates the seizure itself. *Blue arrow* indicates the immediate post-ictal stage

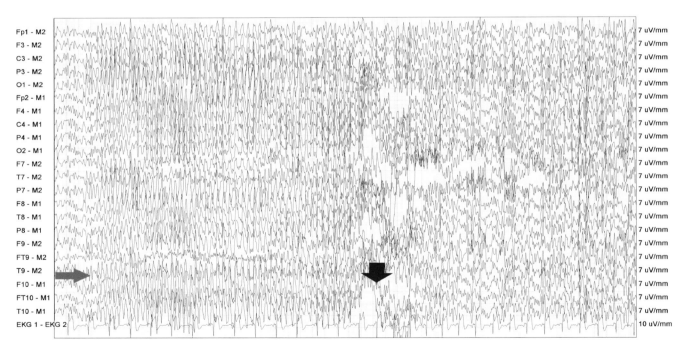

Fig. 4.37 Same epoch as in Fig. 4.36 with a full-head EEG montage. Red arrow indicates the seizure itself. *Blue arrow* indicates the immediate post-ictal stage

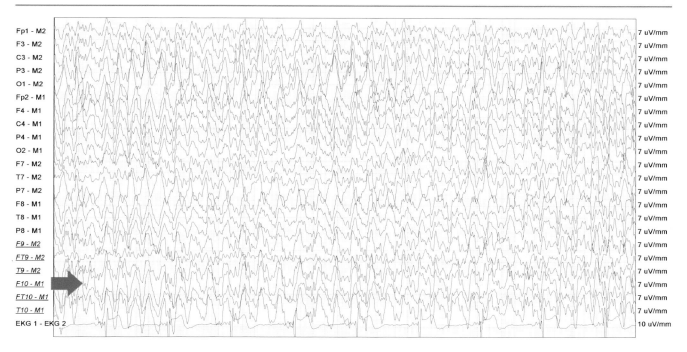

Fig. 4.38 A 10-s portion of Fig. 4.37 at the faster 30 mm/s speed. *Red arrow* indicates the onset of seizure

References

1. Loddenkemper T, Sanchez Fernandez I, Peters JM. Continuous spike and waves during sleep and electrical status epilepticus in sleep. J Clin Neurophysiol. 2011;28:154–64.
2. Tsiptsios DI, Howard RS, Koutroumanidis MA. Electroencephalographic assessment of patients with epileptic seizures. Expert Rev Neurother. 2010;10:1869–86.
3. Hughes JR. Periodic lateralized epileptiform discharges: do they represent an ictal pattern requiring treatment? Epilepsy Behav. 2010;18:162–5.
4. Verma A, Radtke R. EEG of partial seizures. J Clin Neurophysiol. 2006;23:333–9.

Artifacts

5

Keywords

Electrode pop • 60 Hz electrical artifact • Eye movement artifact • Fake eye artifact • Glossokinetic artifact • Grinding • Swallowing artifact • Respiratory artifact • ECG artifact • Sweat artifact • EMG artifact • Body rocking

Artifacts in electroencephalography (EEG) are electrical potentials of nonbrain origin that may be challenging to interpret. Artifacts can be physiological in origin (i.e., derived from electrophysiological properties of other organs) or they can be nonphysiological, resulting from electrical activity of environmental origin. This chapter describes two nonphysiological artifacts and nine physiological sources commonly encountered in EEG.

Electrode Pop

Faulty electrodes, often due to high impedance at the electrode/patient interface, can resemble a spike discharge. Unlike an epileptic discharge, they lack a field, are not followed by slowing, are shorter in duration, and are confined to one electrode [1] (Figs. 5.1–5.4).

Alternating Current Artifact

Also known as 60 Hz in North America and 50 Hz in Europe, alternating current (AC) artifact is generated by the frequency of the alternating pattern of the electrical current and picked up by a loose electrode or one with high impedance [1] (Figs. 5.5–5.10).

Eye Movement Artifact

The eye, like most biological tissues, contains an electrical dipole. The cornea is electropositive and the retina electronegative; therefore, eye movements create electric signals sometimes captured in EEG channels [1] (Figs. 5.11–5.16).

Glossokinetic Artifact

Glossokinetic (tongue) movements may cause significant artifacts in the EEG. The tongue, like the eye, is a bioelectric dipole, with the root of the tongue positive relative to the tip [1]. These movements can be seen in patients in oral dyskinesias, such as palatal myoclonus, and do not resolve in sleep (Figs. 5.17–5.19).

Teeth-Grinding Artifact

Bruxism (teeth grinding) can present with sudden bursts of intense myogenic or muscle artifact (Figs. 5.20–5.22).

H.P. Attarian and N.S. Undevia, *Atlas of Electroencephalography in Sleep Medicine*, DOI 10.1007/978-1-4614-2293-8_5, © Springer Science+Business Media, LLC 2012

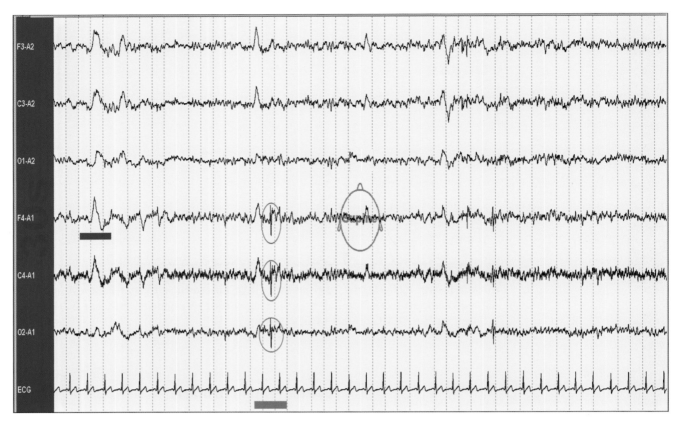

Fig. 5.1 A pop appears as a positive (down-going) waveform (*circled in red*) in all channels using A1 as a reference. *Red bar* highlights the QRS complex of the electrocardiography (ECG). Note how the sharp wave of the pop is not lining up with the QRS, making this not an ECG artifact. *Blue bar* underlines a K complex, indicating that this is an epoch of N2 sleep

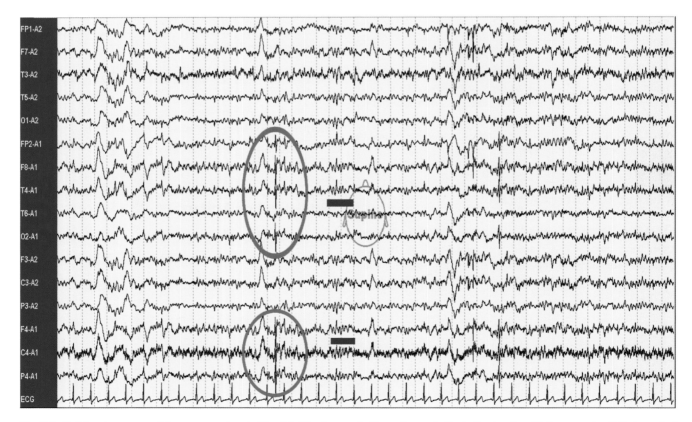

Fig. 5.2 Full-head montage of the same epoch as in Fig. 5.1. *Blue bars* underline a sleep spindle, indicating that this is an epoch of N2 sleep. *Red circles* indicate a pop at the A1 electrode

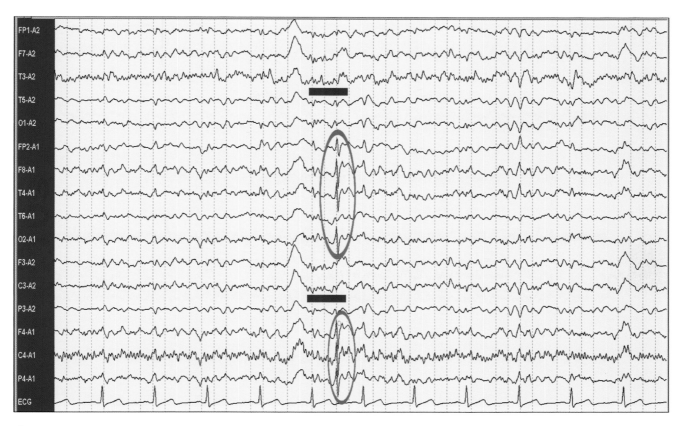

Fig. 5.3 A 10-s window of the same epoch as in Fig. 5.2 at 30 mm/s speed. *Blue bars* underline a sleep spindle, indicating that this is an epoch of N2 sleep. *Red circles* indicate pop at the A1 electrode

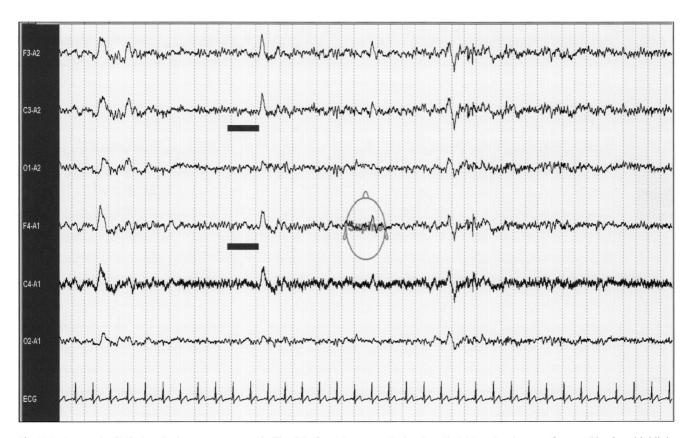

Fig. 5.4 An epoch of N2 sleep in the same person as in Fig. 5.3 after A1 was regelled and applied. Note the absence of a pop. *Blue bars* highlight the sleep spindles

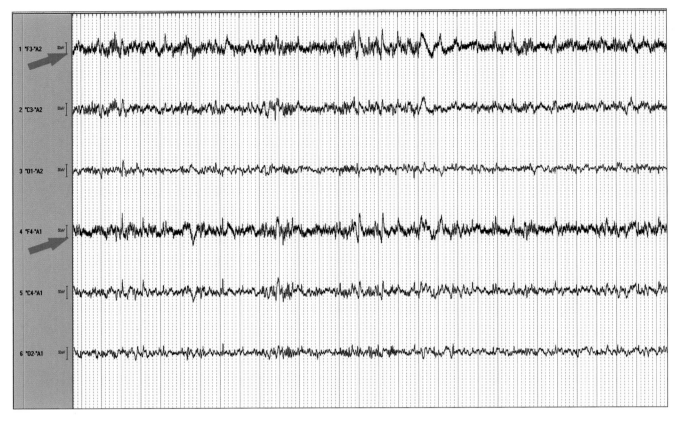

Fig. 5.5 *Red arrows* indicate channels marred by a very fast overlay of activity that blurs the underlying EEG. This is characteristic of an AC artifact

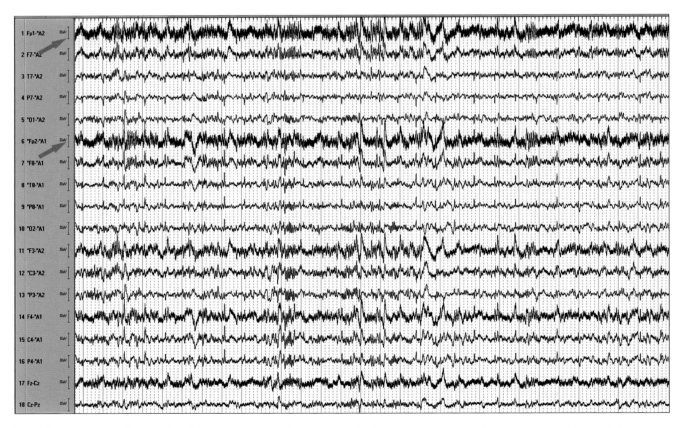

Fig. 5.6 The same N2 sleep epoch as in Fig. 5.5 with a full-head montage. *Red arrows* indicate channels marred by the 60-Hz artifact

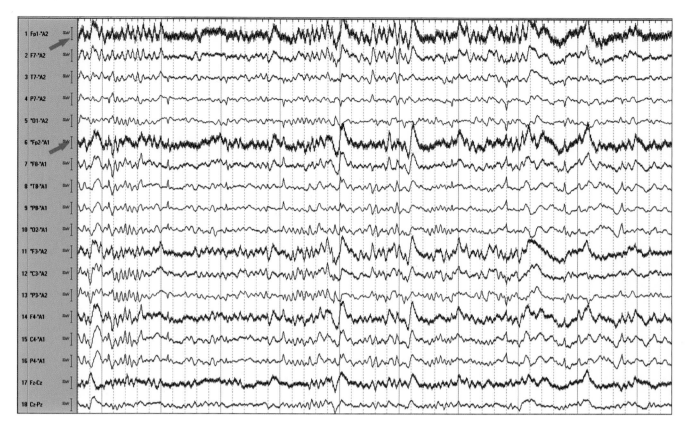

Fig. 5.7 A 10-s window of the same epoch as in Fig. 5.6 at 30 mm/s speed. *Red arrows* indicate channels marred by the 60-Hz artifact

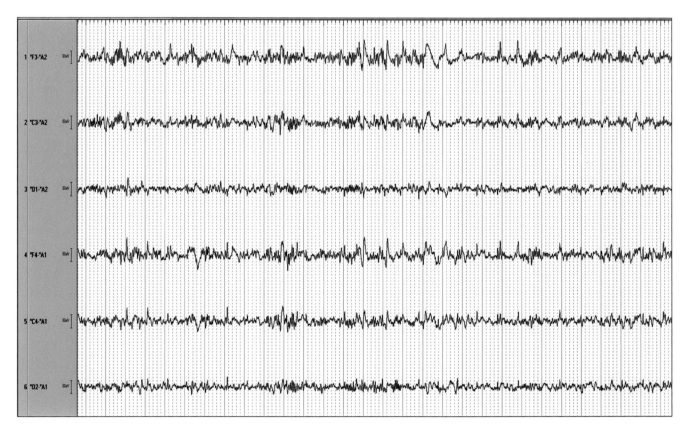

Fig. 5.8 Polysomnography (PSG) epoch described in Fig. 5.7 with the notch (60 Hz) filter applied which removes this artifact. Note how clearly the spindles appear once the electrical artifact is eliminated

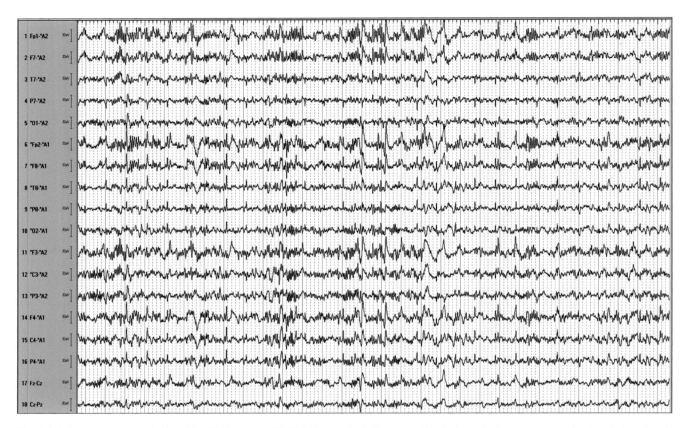

Fig. 5.9 The same epoch as in Fig. 5.8 with the notch (60 Hz) filter applied. Note how clearly the spindles appear once the electrical artifact is eliminated

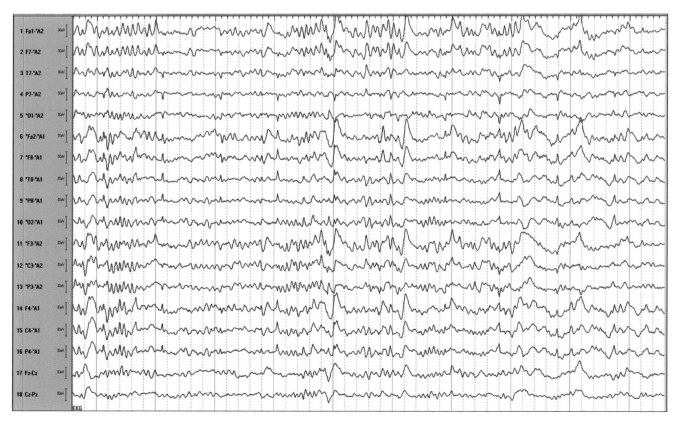

Fig. 5.10 The same epoch as in Fig. 5.9 with the notch (60 Hz) filter applied. Note how clearly the spindles appear once the electrical artifact is eliminated

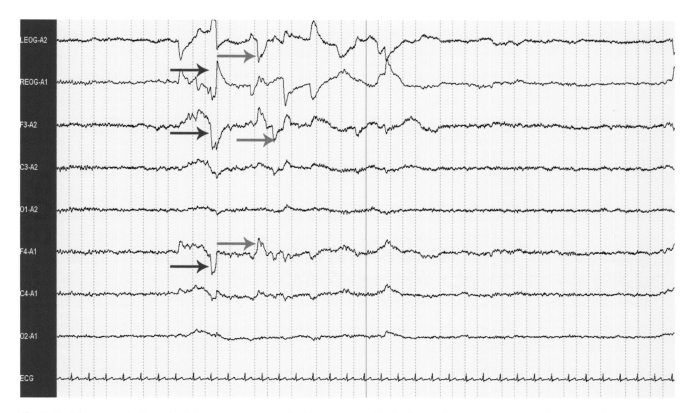

Fig. 5.11 *Blue arrows* indicate the right eye movement and artifacts generated in the frontal channels. *Red arrow* indicates the left eye movement and artifacts generated in the frontal channels

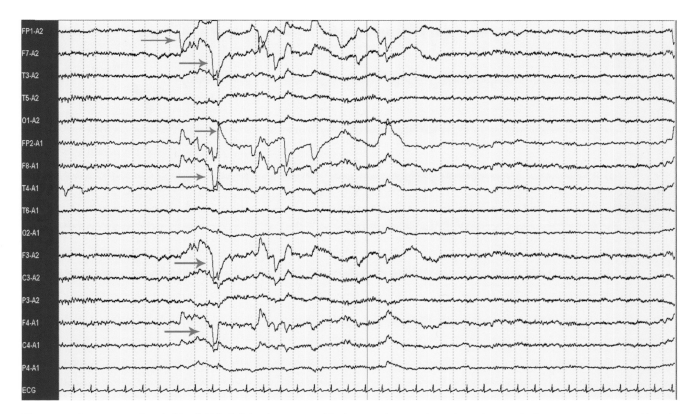

Fig. 5.12 The same epoch as in Fig. 5.11 in full-head montage with electrooculogram channels. *Red arrows* indicate eye movement artifacts in the frontopolar (Fp) and frontal (F) electrodes

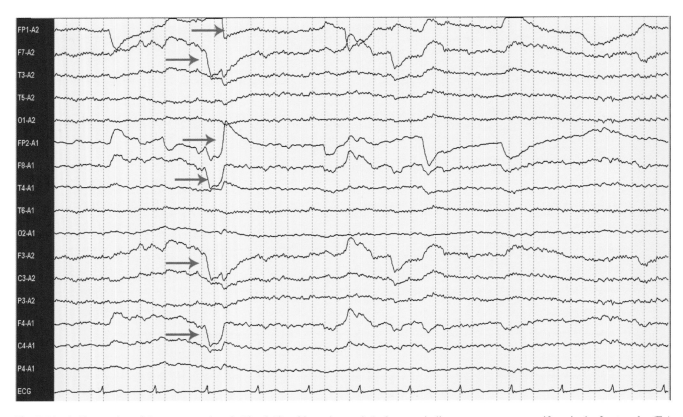

Fig. 5.13 A 10-s portion of the same epoch as in Fig. 5.12 at 30 mm/s speed. *Red arrows* indicate eye movement artifacts in the frontopolar (Fp) and frontal (F) electrodes

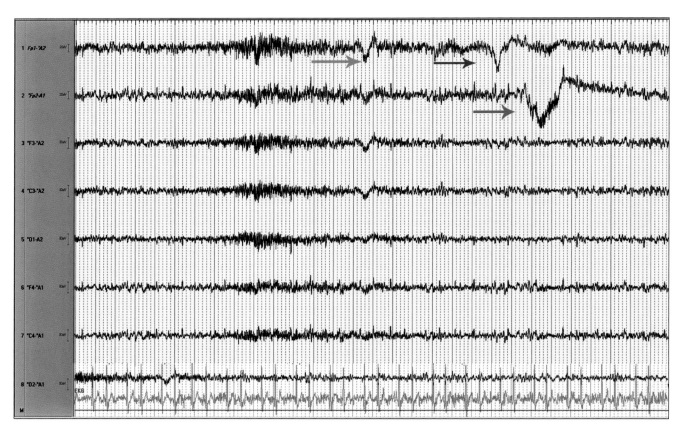

Fig. 5.14 The PSG of a patient with a prosthetic right eye. *Green and blue arrows* indicate eye blink artifacts. *Red arrow* indicates the slower potential generated by the prosthetic eye, although it is not an inherently dipole-generating biological tissue. The polarity of the potential due to eyelid movement is opposite to that due to vertical ocular rotation in the same direction. The potential occurs in the absence of ocular rotation [2]

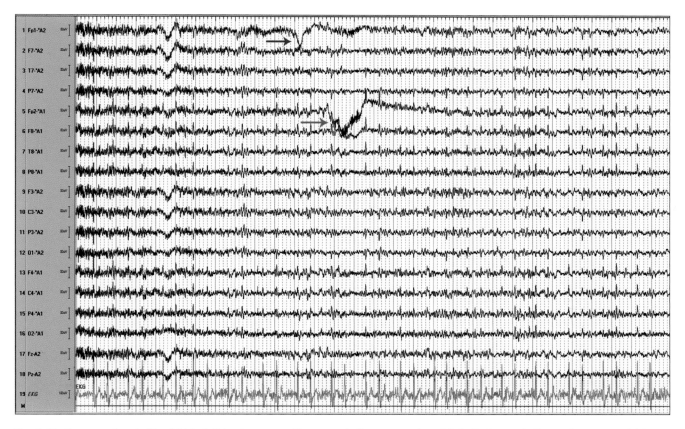

Fig. 5.15 Same epoch as in Fig. 5.14 in full-head montage. *Blue arrow* indicates normal eye blink. *Red arrow* indicates slower potential from a prosthetic eye

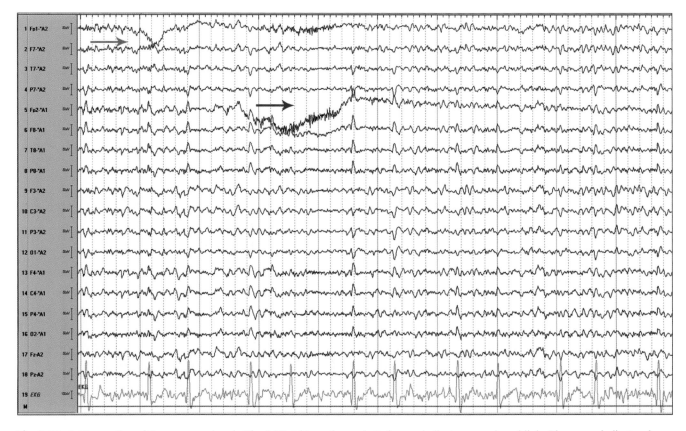

Fig. 5.16 A 10-s portion of the same epoch as in Fig. 5.15 at 30 mm/s speed. *Red arrow* indicates normal eye blink. *Blue arrow* indicates slower potential from a prosthetic eye

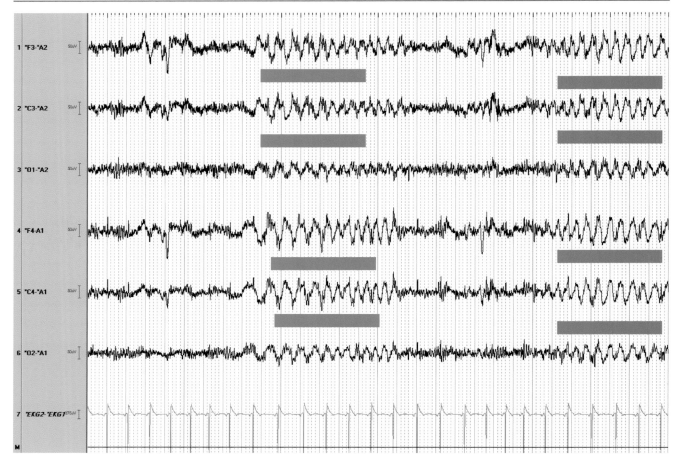

Fig. 5.17 A 30-s epoch of an edentulous patient moving his tongue intermittently as he tries to fall asleep. *Red bars* underline the glossokinetic artifact

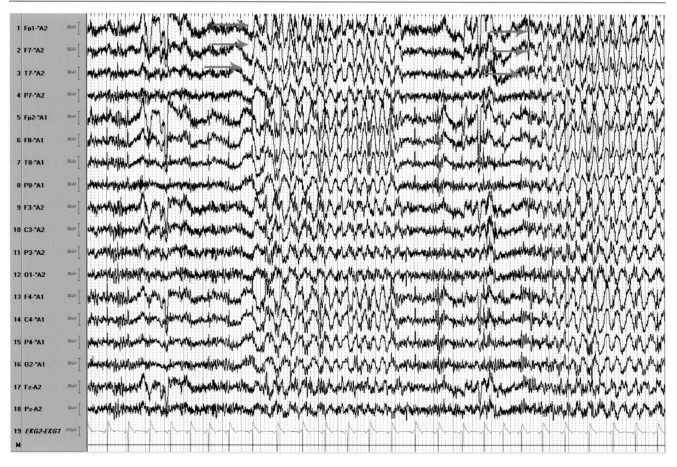

Fig. 5.18 The same epoch as in Fig. 5.17 in a full-head montage. *Red arrows* indicate the glossokinetic artifact. As seen here, the artifact is greatest in the frontal and temporal derivations

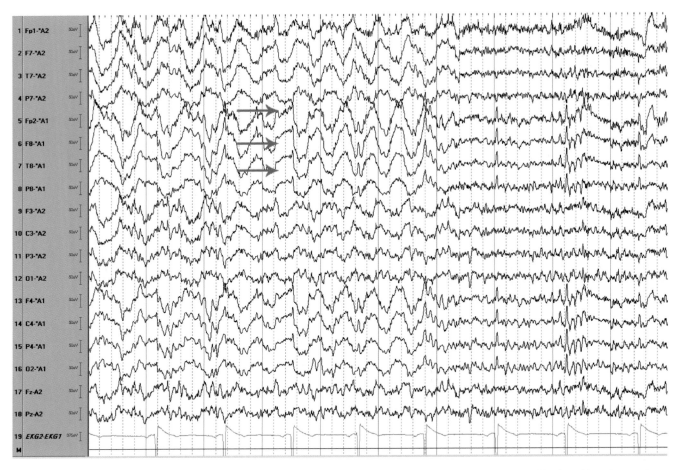

Fig. 5.19 A 10-s portion of the same epoch as in Fig. 5.18 at 30 mm/s paper speed. *Red arrows* indicate the glossokinetic artifact. As seen here, the artifact is usually greatest in the frontal and temporal derivations

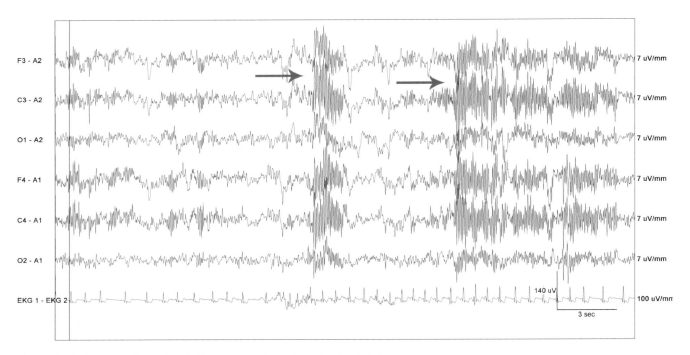

Fig. 5.20 *Red arrows* indicate the grinding artifact. The patient is in stage N2 sleep

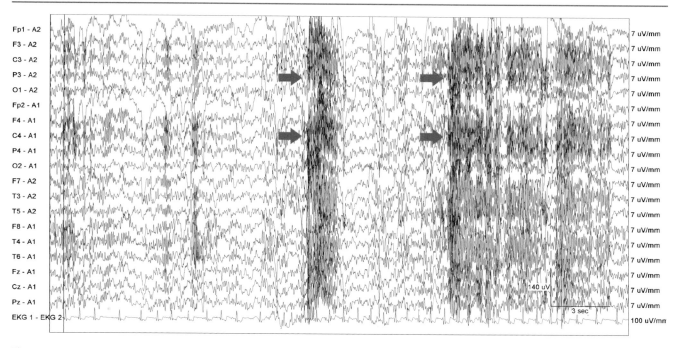

Fig. 5.21 The same epoch as in Fig. 5.20 in a full-EEG montage. *Red arrows* again indicate the grinding artifact. Note how the underlying EEG is obscured by the intensity of the muscle activity

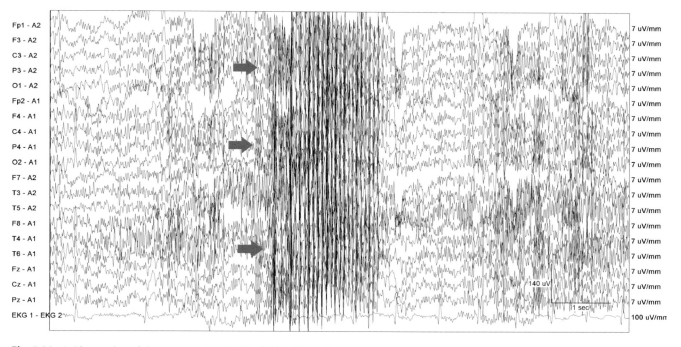

Fig. 5.22 A 10-s portion of the same epoch as in Fig. 5.21 at 30 mm/s paper speed. *Red arrows* indicate the grinding artifact

Swallowing Artifact

Because of the number of facial and cranial muscles used during swallowing, this particular artifact usually consists of a brief rhythmic slow activity generated by the tongue with an overlay of very sharp myogenic artifact [1] (Figs. 5.23–5.25).

Respiratory Artifact

This is an important artifact to identify in polysomnography and an easy one as we routinely monitor breathing parameters during sleep studies (Figs. 5.26–5.28).

Electrocardiographic Artifact

ECG artifact can mimic periodic epileptiform discharges on EEG because of its rhythmicity [1] (Figs. 5.29–5.31).

Sweat Artifact

Sweat artifact has a very slow (0.25–0.50 Hz) and characteristic appearance that is readily identifiable by its wavering baseline [1] (Figs. 5.32–5.34).

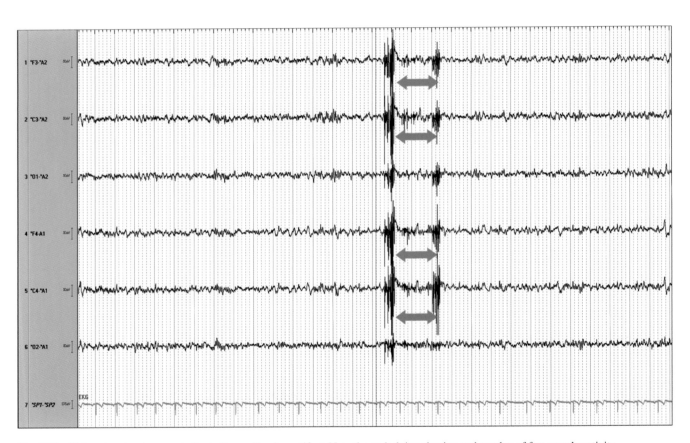

Fig. 5.23 *Bidirectional red arrows* indicate the swallowing artifact. Note the underlying slowing and overlay of fast muscle activity

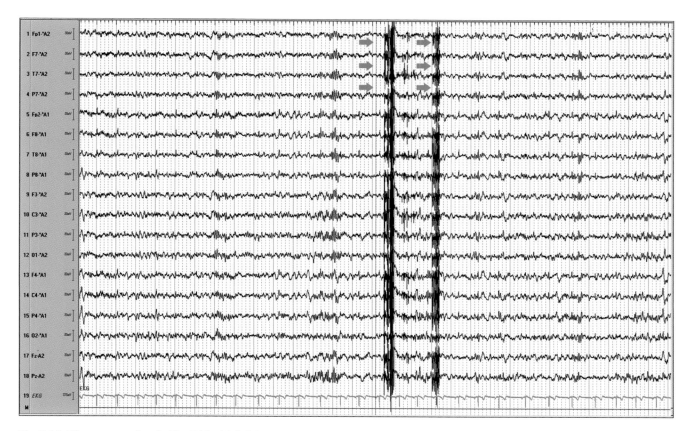

Fig. 5.24 The same epoch as in Fig. 5.23 with full-head montage. *Red arrows* indicate the swallowing artifact. Note the underlying slowing and the overlay of fast muscle activity

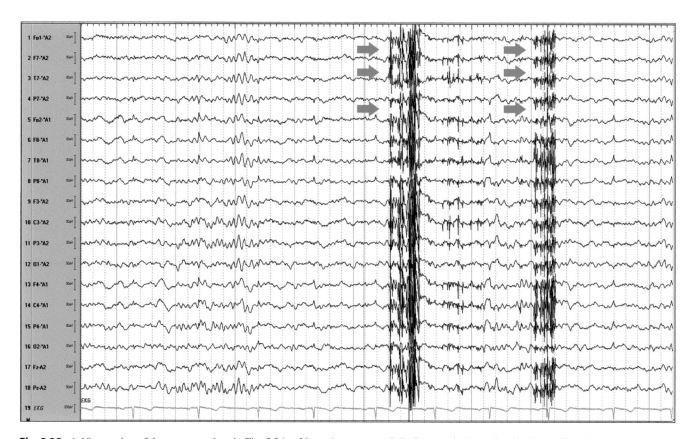

Fig. 5.25 A 10-s portion of the same epoch as in Fig. 5.24 at 30 mm/s paper speed. *Red arrows* indicate the grinding artifact. Note the underlying slowing (clearer at this paper speed) and the overlay of fast muscle activity

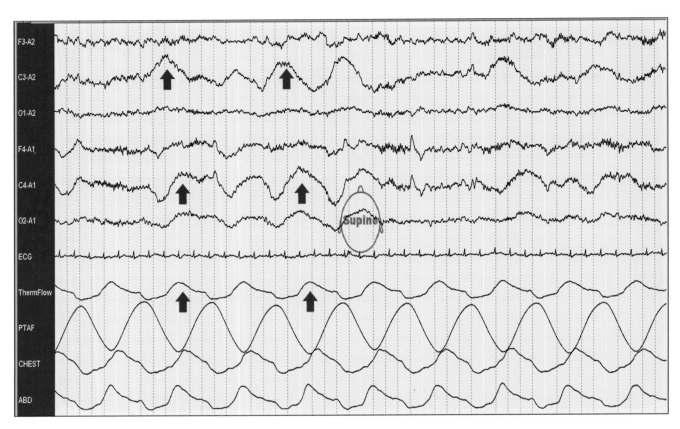

Fig. 5.26 *Blue arrows* indicate the respiratory artifact in the EEG channels. Note how they are time-synced to the breathing signals in the respiratory channels

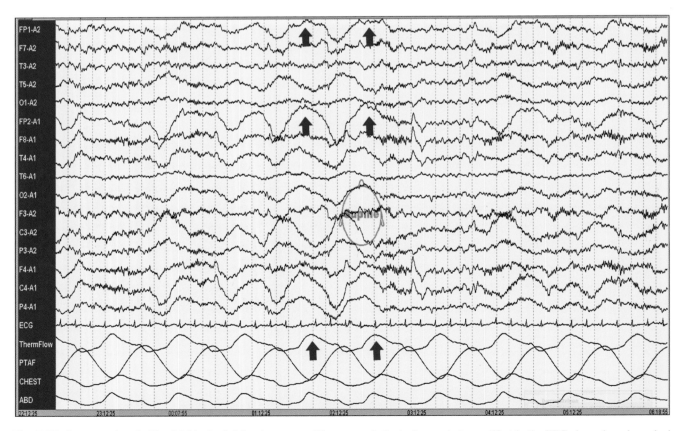

Fig. 5.27 Same epoch as in Fig. 5.26 in the full-head montage. *Blue arrows* indicate the respiratory artifact in the EEG channels and synched breathing signals in the respiratory channels

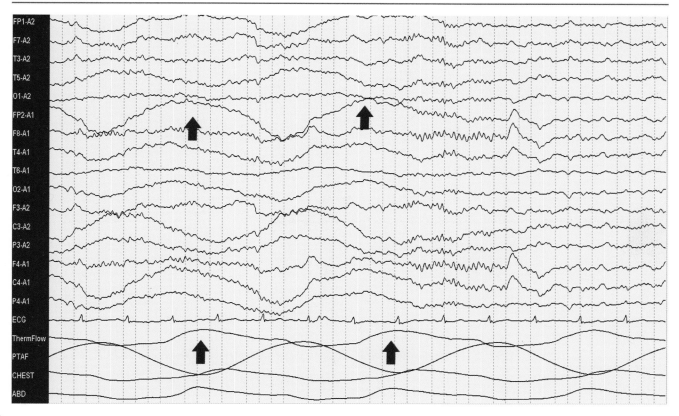

Fig. 5.28 A 10-s portion of the same epoch as in Fig. 5.28 at 30 mm/s paper speed. *Blue arrows* indicate the respiratory artifact in the EEG channels and synched breathing signals in the respiratory channels

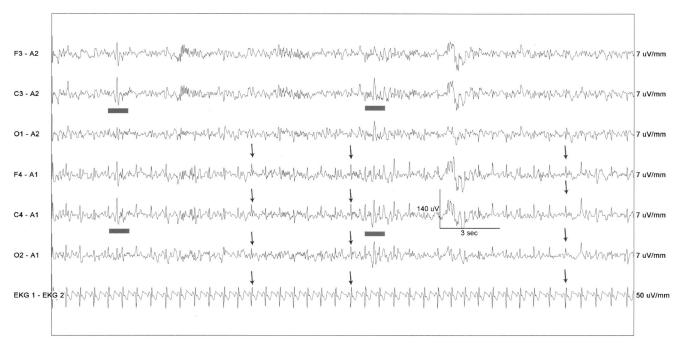

Fig. 5.29 To help differentiate an ECG artifact from epileptiform discharges, this is the PSG of a patient who has both. The ECG artifact (*blue arrows*) is sharper, smaller in amplitude, and time synched to the ECG channel activity. *Red bars* underline the epileptiform discharges that are higher amplitude and maximal at the central leads

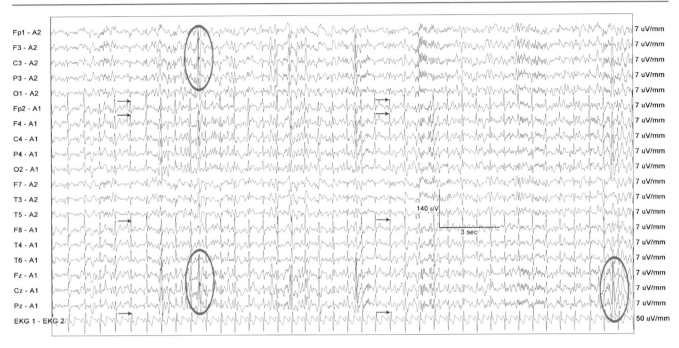

Fig. 5.30 Same epoch as in Fig. 5.29 in the full-head montage. *Red ovals* highlight the epileptiform discharges maximal at C3. *Blue arrows* point to the ECG artifact

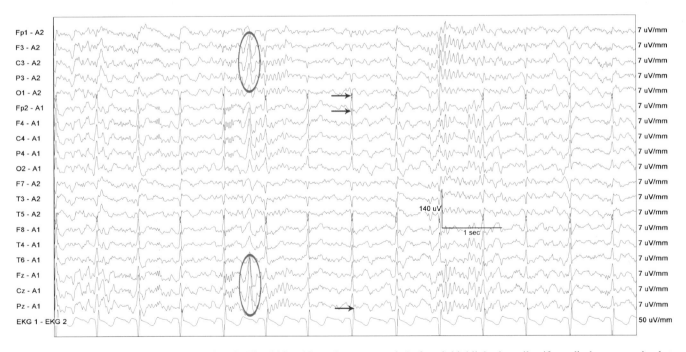

Fig. 5.31 A 10-s portion of the same epoch as in Fig. 5.30 at 30 mm/s paper speed. *Red ovals* highlight the epileptiform discharges maximal at C3. *Blue arrows* indicate the ECG artifact

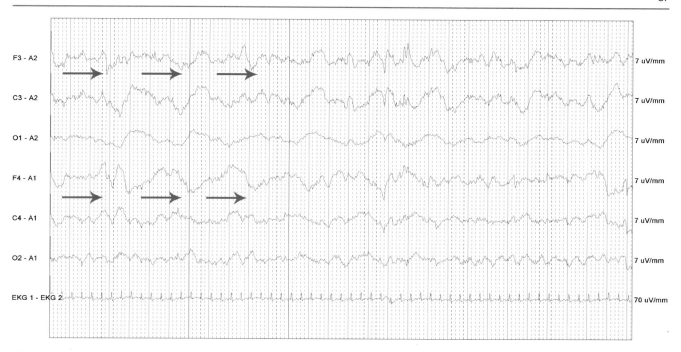

Fig. 5.32 *Red arrows* indicate the sweat artifact. Note the wavering baseline and characteristic slow frequency of the artifact

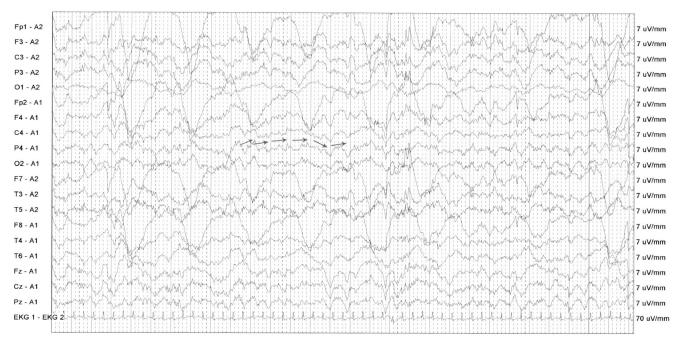

Fig. 5.33 Same epoch as in Fig. 5.32 in full-head montage. *Red arrows* indicate the artifact

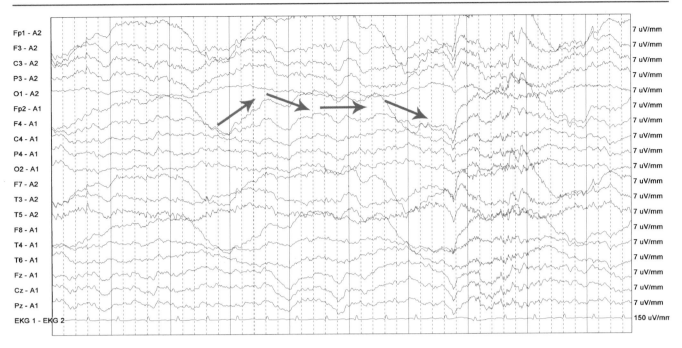

Fig. 5.34 A 10-s portion of the same epoch as in Fig. 5.33 at 30 mm/s paper speed. *Red arrows* indicate the artifact

Myogenic Artifact

Myogenic [muscle or electromyography (EMG)] artifact is the most commonly observed artifact on EEG. The temporalis and frontalis muscles are the two main producers of this artifact [1]. This is often noted earlier in the polysomnography recording and resolves as the patient relaxes once asleep (Figs. 5.35–5.37).

Body Rocking Artifact

This is a complex movement artifact seen usually in patients undergoing PSG and suffering from a sleep rhythmic movement disorder (SRMD). Use of additional electrodes helps define this type of artifact [3] (Figs. 5.38–5.41).

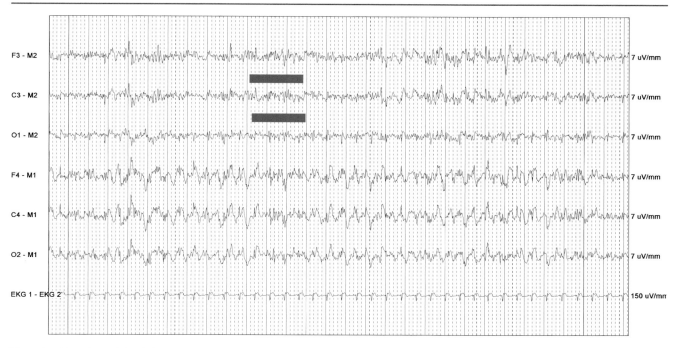

Fig. 5.35 Note the *red* highlighted channels that demonstrate fast, low-amplitude, EMG activity, overlaying the EEG primarily in the left frontal and central channels

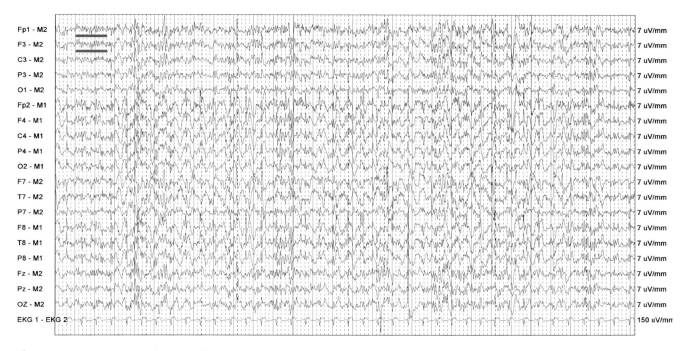

Fig. 5.36 Same epoch as in Fig. 5.35 in full-head montage. Note the *red* highlighted channels that demonstrate fast, low-amplitude EMG activity overlaying the EEG primarily in the left frontal and central channels

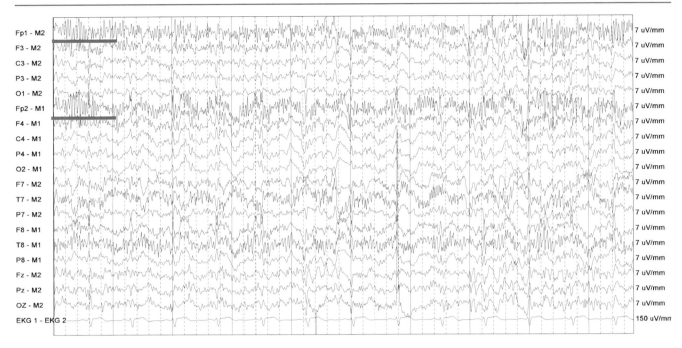

Fig. 5.37 A 10-s portion of the same epoch as in Fig. 5.36 at 30 mm/s paper speed. *Red bars* underline the EMG artifact in the frontopolar channels. Note that increasing the paper speed more clearly differentiates the EMG and EEG

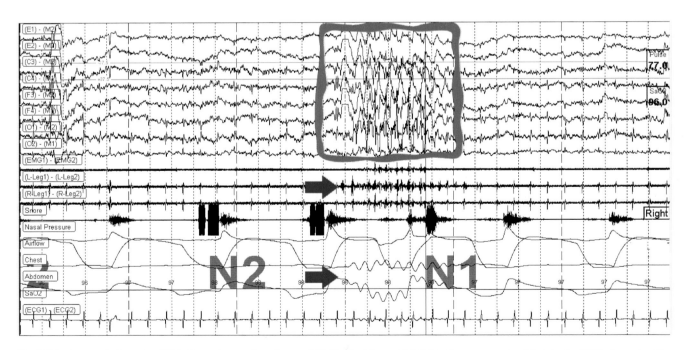

Fig. 5.38 An epoch from the PSG of a patient undergoing an SRMD. *Red frame* highlights the movement artifact in the EEG channels. *Blue arrows* indicate the increased EMG activity in the leg leads

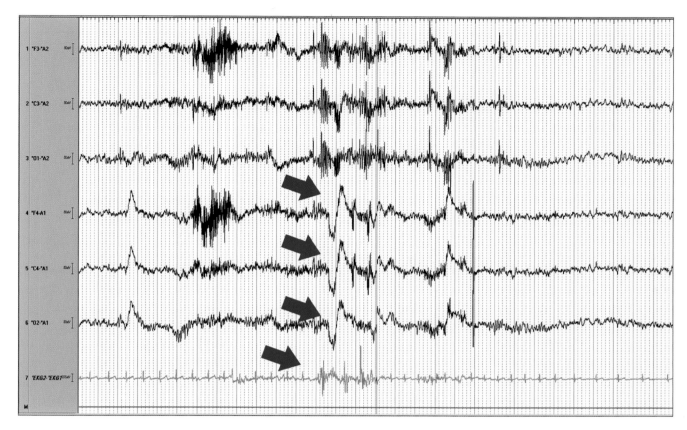

Fig. 5.39 An epoch from another patient with SRMD, although one with a less dramatic event. *Blue arrows* indicate the movement artifact seen mainly on the right with an overlay of heavy myogenic artifact

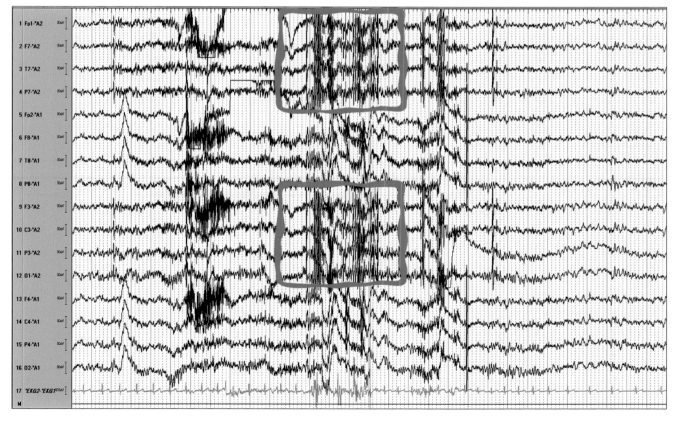

Fig. 5.40 Same epoch as in Fig. 5.39 in full montage. *Red frames* highlight the movement artifact in the EEG channels with an overlay of heavy myogenic artifact

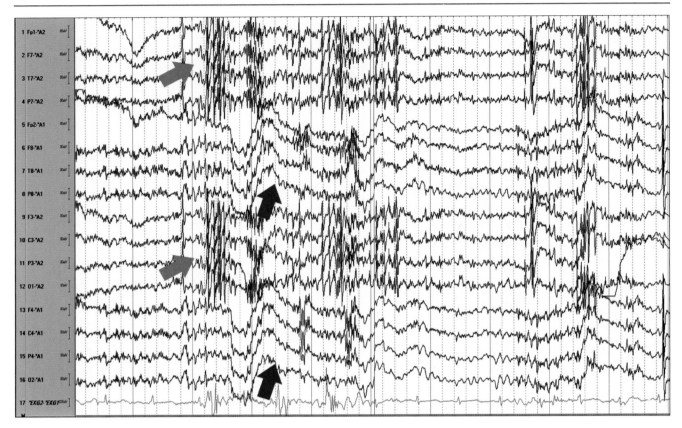

Fig. 5.41 A 10-s portion of the same epoch as in Fig. 5.40 at 30 mm/s paper speed. *Blue arrows* indicate the movement artifact and *red arrows* indicate the EMG artifact

References

1. Tatum WO, Dworetzky BA, Schomer DL. Artifact and recording concepts in EEG. J Clin Neurophysiol. 2011;28:252–63.

2. Matsuo F, Shaner EE. EEG artifact due to a metallic prosthetic eye. Am J EEG Technol. 1975;15:75–8.

3. Tatum WO, Dworetzky BA, Freeman WD, Schomer DL. Artifact: recording EEG in special care units. J Clin Neurophysiol. 2011; 28:264–7.

Index